THE GOOD SEX BIBLE

A Committed Couples' Guide to Keeping Relationships Lively, Intimate and Gratifying

First Edition

Daniel Beaver

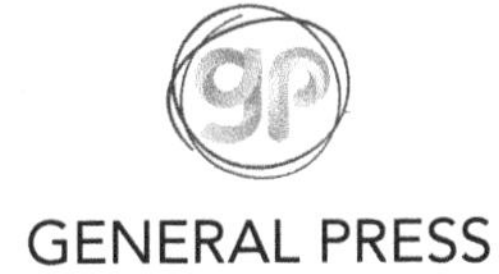

GENERAL PRESS

Published in India by

GENERAL PRESS

4228/1, Ansari Road, Daryaganj, New Delhi 110002
Ph: (011) 23282971, 45795759
Email: generalpressindia@gmail.com
www.generalpress.in

First Published in the United States by

COGNELLA INC.

3970 Sorrento Valley Blvd
San Diego, CA 92121, USA

The Good Sex Bible
By Daniel Beaver
First Indian Edition : 2017
ISBN : 9788180320224

THIS EDITION IS FOR SALE IN INDIA ONLY.

Contents

This book is dedicated to Nancy, the most sensuous woman I have ever loved. You truly are an inspiration to my life. Without you, writing this book would have been difficult. You are my best friend, my only and best lover, and my lovely wife. Thanks for being in my life. I am truly blessed, and I love you.

Preface

Virtually everyone I talk to wants a satisfying and fulfilling sex life, and this is particularly true of married couples. But is this goal being attained? I think not. As a culture, we may seem preoccupied with sex—given the media's emphasis on the way we look and perform—but what we see on television and the Internet doesn't necessarily reflect what really goes on in our bedrooms.

A disparity still exists between what couples want and what they experience in their daily lives. This conflict between expectation and reality causes a great deal of frustration and resentment that spills over into other aspects of people's lives. When I first presented my agent with the idea for this book, he felt that a book about sex would be more marketable than one about marriage. Sex sells! It sells because we have an unfulfilled need for quality in our sex lives. We try to get this need met in all kinds of ways, through books, therapy, and the all-knowing Internet. We as a culture are looking for anything that might help us in our quest for the magic key to a fulfilling sex life.

Why another book about sex? So far, I haven't seen a book that addresses the issue of sexuality in the context of a committed couple's relationship in a way that the layperson can understand, and to which he or she can relate. True, the subject of sex in popular literature has been thoroughly dissected in books, videos, and the Internet—on female sexuality, male sexuality, orgasms, the G-spot, and so on and on—but a person needs an entire library in order to look at the whole picture as opposed to all the parts. One of my intentions in writing this book, therefore, is to offer a comprehensive package of information that deals with what really happens psychologically in a couple's sexual relationship. The issue, as I see it, is quality—the amount of pleasure, satisfaction, intimacy, and fulfillment that people experience in their sex lives.

This is my third book (part of a triad) dealing with the overall subject of intimacy. My previous book, *Creating the Intimate Connection*, explores how a couple can have greater intimacy outside the bedroom—how they can intimately communicate with one another on an intimate level, and how they can resolve conflicts within the context of a committed relationship. Without emotional intimacy, true sexual intimacy would be difficult, if not impossible. The third part of the triad is my book, *Learning to Love Yourself: The First Step in Having a Successful Relationship*. I highly recommend that you read the first two books before this one.

In my therapy practice, before I look at a couple's sexual relationship, I make sure that their general relationship is sound, that their conflicts are resolved, and that they are able to talk to each other intimately. They need to be lovers outside the bedroom before they can experience a quality sexual relationship in the bedroom. I think that too often the subject of sex is taken out of the context of the whole relationship, and we forget that our sexuality is more than what we do in bed.

Some people ask, "Why should there have to be books, classes, and therapies devoted to sex in the first place? Isn't sex a natural function that doesn't require any learning or teaching? If left alone, won't nature take care of it on its own?" Many people are surprised to learn that the only natural (i.e., instinctual, not requiring learning) thing about sex is the actual process of making babies, or reproduction. In principle, this aspect of sexuality doesn't require a great deal of knowledge and intelligence. Ironically, this is really the only aspect of sexuality that we do learn about in our culture. By the time I graduated from high school, I knew how babies were made. But I didn't know how to enjoy making love to a woman. Everything I learned from parents, church, schools, and peers about pleasurable sexuality was in some way repressive; all the mixed messages, guilt trips, and fears that I inherited from these sources inhibited or repressed my so-called natural ability to enjoy the sexual experience. This suggests that sex might be a naturally pleasurable and fulfilling experience in this culture if we weren't taught all the dos and don'ts that inhibit us! My generation used drugs, both alcohol and marijuana, to chemically liberate us from all the antipleasure messages we received. I would like to liberate people psychologically without having to resort to chemicals.

The emphasis of this book is on the aspects of sexuality that we are never taught—how to achieve maximum pleasure in our sexual lives and how to maintain the quality of pleasure over a long period of time. In our culture, this requires a type of sex education we never had. From my vantage point being a part of the upper education system, things haven't changed, even with the invention of the Internet, which provides an abundance of information on the topic of sex.

The way we learn about the actual dynamics of sex between two people is through firsthand experience, which really means that we learn about sex through trial and error—unfortunately, mostly through error. Something as vitally important, as personal, and as sensitive as our sexual life we leave to fumbling around in the dark. Is it any wonder that we have so many hang-ups and fears about our sexual experience? And these feelings severely limit our ability to enjoy our full sexual potential.

Sex is a natural drive in all of us—just like hunger and thirst—though unlike these latter drives, our sexuality can be repressed without fatal consequences. Everyone is a sexual person. Even those who seem to have no desire for sex have a potential to be very sexual. The challenge is to break through all the conditioning and inhibiting experiences that get in the way of enjoying our full sexual capability. It is my intention through this book to show how to break through the psychological traps to which we all may fall prey, which get in the way of experiencing full sexual pleasure and fulfillment.

The main context for my discussion of sexuality will be that of the married couple, since marital sex is the most widely approved form of sexuality in our culture, since the majority of people marry, and also since most of my clinical experience has been gained from working with married couples. However, most of this material will be relevant to the single person, the couple living together, or homosexual couples, legally married or not.

One might think that since marriage is the most common context for sexual activity, marital sex must therefore be usually pleasurable and fulfilling. Yet, just the contrary is true. Sex tends to occur less and less frequently through the course of a marriage. All around us, we hear a constant outcry about the quality of sex in marriage and about the quality of marriage in general. Renowned sex therapists William Masters and Virginia Johnson suggest that half of all marriages involve some sexual dysfunction.

Any discussion of sexuality in this culture is bound to be emotionally charged. We are dealing with people's values of right and wrong, morality and immorality. My intent is to stay clear of moral issues. I respect everyone's values—who am I to judge? If a person's beliefs work, and the person's values, beliefs, and attitudes are not working and are interfering with their sexual life, then I can offer some alternative ways of thinking and acting that may help them to enjoy more sexual satisfaction and fulfillment in their personal life.

Examples and references used in this book are based on actual situations I've encountered in counseling, but in some instances, the cases described are composites of several actual cases. In all cases, the names and details of each person have been changed.

–Daniel Beaver, MS, MFT

Introduction

When I first wrote The Good Sex Bible it was 1990. At that time, I wanted to write a book that reflected the work I was doing with couples in the context of sex therapy. This clinical work was greatly influenced by the training I received by a team of therapists who worked with Dr. William Masters and Virginia Johnson 16 years earlier.

A lot has changed in the area of human sexuality since 1990, and I realized that there was much more new information I was teaching in my Human Sexuality college classes. In addition, there were new issues I was addressing in my clinical practice. As a result of these changes, I felt it was time to write an updated version of The Good Sex Bible.

The first big change has been the influence of the Internet in our daily lives, but for the purposes of this book, its influence on our sexual lives has created some profound differences. I will try to address what is relevant.

The other major change has been the development of erectile dysfunction medications. In 1990, no one had heard of medications like Viagra or Cialis. These drugs have had a major influence on how I treat erectile dysfunction with patients seeking my therapeutic help, making earlier forms of treatment somewhat obsolete for certain patients. It became embarrassing that these medications weren't present in my first edition of The Good Sex Bible.

Other changes that are added to this new edition are subjects I lectured about in my college classes, but weren't included in my first edition of the book. These new chapters include a new, expanded version of sex and history; sexual development; sociological influence on our sexual development; a chapter on sexual anatomy; and one on sexual physiology.

In this new edition, I attempted to bring more of my own personal and professional experience to this book. This comes with living longer, and as a result, I have a lot more information to share. I hope this makes the book less clinical and academic sounding. Now, after 40 years of clinical and academic experience in the area of sexuality, my perspective on the subject is richer and broader than it was back in 1990.

Often, when I address groups or teaching classes on the subject of sexuality and relationships, invariably, I'm asked how I became a sex therapist. How did I seek out this specialty in addition to the more traditional forms of counseling and therapy?

My answer is always the same. It was not at all something I planned—perhaps fate played a big part in my choice. Certain doors opened up to me that I really wouldn't have known were there unless I had recognized the opportunity and walked through them.

I began my career in marriage and family therapy, taking a job with a family service agency soon after earning my master's degree in counseling. I had not been with the agency long when the executive director took me aside and asked if I would consider attending a training class offered by the California Department of Public Health. It was entitled, "Team Treatment to Couple Counseling."

The training program would be three months long, I was told, and I would get my full salary while attending, in addition to picking up some necessary professional training. I jumped at the chance, even before I'd explored what material was going to be covered.

To my surprise (and the surprise of the executive director), the course turned out to be Masters and Johnson sex therapy training. Over the next 90 days, I received the first real sex education of my life, both from a personal and professional point of view.

My previous sex education was pretty limited. I got the basic facts of reproduction from my junior high school gym coach. This sex education consisted of a week of lectures in a health and hygiene class on the dangers of drugs, sexually transmitted diseases (what they called VD, or venereal disease, in those days), followed by a discussion on sex. In high school, I had a follow-up course, this time taught by a young woman who was anything but comfortable talking about sex with a bunch of sweaty-palmed coeds.

In my first year at college, I became interested in looking at Masters and Johnson's new book, *The Human Sexual Response*. This might have been an early foreshadowing of my coming career. When I went to the school library to look at the book, I discovered it was kept locked in a glass cabinet. The librarian in charge of this cabinet was an elderly woman who guarded the books sequestered there as if they were top secret—delicate material not meant for the average library goer. Whatever spirit had moved me to read this book was dampened by the prospect of having to pass muster with the keeper of the keys.

I took many psychology classes at the University of California, but there was only a single class offered on sexuality. It dealt with the sex life of beagles. While this might have been invaluable had I been interested in a career in veterinary medicine, I decided it wasn't for me.

It was from this grossly limited background in human sexuality that I entered the Masters and Johnson course. And it was here that I had to face the fact that I was only slightly more comfortable with the subject than the keeper of the keys in the college library. During the three-month course, I learned to use language and talk about subjects I had never before imagined. I had to work through some of my own misinformation about sex and confront what was uncomfortable to me. Upon completion of the course, I had a brand-new outlook, not only about sexuality itself, but about my own life and the meaning of having a long-term intimate relationship.

If this course awakened me to the role of sexuality in human relations, the next step in my sex education helped open me physically. This phase of my learning was also more serendipitous than intentional. Back in the 1970s, I often spoke at human sexuality courses given at the local colleges. On this particular occasion, the instructor, Allure Jeffcoat, had used up her budget for outside speakers, so in return for my presentation to her class, she offered me a weekend massage class that she was teaching.

I agreed to make the trade, not giving too much thought to what it might involve. When I showed up for the class, however, it became quite clear that we were all going to be nude. I had never experienced anything like this in my life, and I had all kinds of illusions run through my mind—not the least of which was that I would keep getting an erection. I was not alone in my discomfort. Others confessed to having similar concerns or being worried about how their bodies would compare to others.

To my surprise, my exaggerated sexual concerns quickly faded. For the most part, people in the group became quite comfortable with their nudity. We learned how to touch and be touched, to give and receive a therapeutic massage. Though sensuous and deeply nurturing, it was not a sexual experience. I left with a new experience of the sensual nature of human life. Not only did this class open up new avenues of self-expression, pleasure, awareness, and communication in my own life, it provided me with new levels of understanding to share with my patients and students.

Over the years, I have integrated with my professional knowledge a wide range of disciplines and skills associated with human sexuality. And like most therapists, I have allowed the lessons from my own life to enrich those received by more formal routes. In this book, I have attempted to bring it all together in a form that is easily accessible for anyone wishing to deepen the enjoyment of sex and thus enrich those most intimate moments that we share with our lovers and mates.

1

The History of Sex Through the Ages

Whenever I meet with a couple for the first time during the sex therapy process, we sit down, and I ask them about their sex history. I ask them about all the experiences in their past that might have had an impact on them in terms of shaping and influencing their sexuality today. From our discussions together, we begin to develop a sympathetic understanding of how their present ideas and feelings about sex and their own self-esteem have come about. In the beginning, many couples are skeptical about this process. To them, events that happened in the past are ancient history. However, after a sexual breakthrough or two, which allows them to experience deeper and more intimate levels of their relationship, they enthusiastically acknowledge the tremendous value of such work.

For each of us, our sexual history is both cultural and personal. What's the difference between the two? Admittedly, there are times when one overlaps into the other. But in general, personal history is the sum of our sexual experiences, while cultural history is comprised of the sexual memories and beliefs of the human race. The latter are passed along to us through our parents, our peers, our schools, the media, and our religious institutions.

Sex Through the Ages

It is often said that if you ignore the past, you are doomed to repeat it. This is true with sexual history, because when you look at the sexual history of Western civilization, there are many repetitive themes. There are also cycles that tend to flip-flop over time between liberal and conservative periods.

My approach to this section is just to give you the highlights of each historical period as it relates to the cultural sexuality of the time and how that might be relevant to us today. One could write volumes of material regarding the sexual history of mankind, but in this chapter, I just want to give you a very superficial level of the historical sexual past of Western civilization.

The Greek and Roman Periods

The first period of history I will start with is the time of the ancient Greeks and Romans. This period was the most sexually open and uninhibited period in Western civilization. In ancient Greece, sexual themes were prominent parts of the theater and poetry. Many Roman writers also took an open and bawdy approach to sex. The openness about sex in the literature of the Greeks and the Romans reflects their general acceptance of human sexuality.

The Romans basically accepted almost every form or type of sexuality you could think of. Homosexuality, bisexuality, group sex, and adultery were just some of the options. Certain Roman emperors were more outlandish than others; one of the most notorious was the Emperor Caligula. The Romans had public baths; some of them are still preserved in Bath, England.

The Romans believed that their lives were governed by a multitude of gods for different aspects of their lives. So, if the gods didn't strike them down, then whatever they were doing was acceptable. In other words, they had no defined rules about sexual behavior. That didn't mean that mortal man didn't intercede in behaviors they didn't like, such as your neighbor having sex with your wife. You might go and kill your neighbor for "messing around" with her.

The Jews and the Romans

As the Romans expanded their empire, taking over different countries and peoples, they ran into different cultures. They took over the land of Judaea and its people, the Jews. Today, Judaea is part of modern-day Israel. The Jews practiced their own religion, known as Judaism. This religion only had one god, as compared to the many different gods of the Romans. Judaism also was based on a set of rules of behavior for the way people were supposed to conduct their daily lives. These rules were called the Ten Commandments, which were handed down from their one god and given to one of their leaders, Moses.

Judaism was in direct conflict with the way the Romans led their lives; as a result, the Romans weren't too happy with the Jewish people in general. They had a problem with one particular Jewish carpenter from Nazareth known as Jesus Christ, who was going around stirring up the population to make some social changes within the Jewish establishment. I assume most of you know the rest of the story as to what happened to him. Several years after his death on the cross, his disciples started a new religion that separated itself from Judaism, known as Christianity.

The Fall of the Roman Empire

After the demise of the Roman Empire during the 11th century, early Christian traditions and teachings regarding sexuality became more firmly entrenched in Europe. This period is sometimes referred to as the Dark Ages. Life for the common man was short and difficult. The significant concept during this time was that the Church and state were one. Whatever the teachings of the Church were at that time became the law of the land.

The Church's attitude toward sex in general was very oppressive. "The Church had opinions and laws about every aspect of sex. Adultery and fornication in some cases were sins punishable by death, but for a time the Church actually condoned prostitution, admitting that it was a necessary evil. And in the early part of the Middle Ages, priests were actually allowed to marry and have children."(1) The only function of sex was for procreation, a basic theme of historical Christianity. The ruling governments of the time in western Europe followed along in enforcing Church doctrine.

Even though the official attitude of these times was dark and oppressive as it related to sexuality in general, what was occurring with the general population trying to survive in rural areas was quite different. People didn't have a long life expectancy, so they were living more for the moment and didn't pay a lot of attention to the repressive authorities.

The historical theme of having an oppressive sexual overlord—whether the Church or the state—and an active underground occurs repeatedly throughout our journey through the sexual past. Another common historical theme is that a conservative sexual period is usually followed by a very liberal one. The next historical period to follow this trend is known as the Renaissance, which occurred from the 14th to the 18th centuries. The Dark Ages were over.

The Renaissance

Before the Renaissance, sex and sensuality were seen as sins to be repressed. Sex was strictly for reproduction. Religion guarded daily life, and each moment in life was spent on the goal of attaining salvation. After the Black Death, or bubonic plague, in the 14th century, secularism spread, and people were less concerned about salvation and focused more on the enjoyment of their short lifetime.

In the Renaissance, sex and sensuality were seen as the first steps to salvation. It was concluded that love of the body was the first step on the long ladder toward a love of wisdom and ultimately of God, and therefore it was to be embraced and not hidden away.

This period in England started during the reign of Queen Elizabeth I. During this time, the concept of "pure love," or courtly love, developed regarding women among the upper classes. Women were elevated to an immaculate place where romanticism, secrecy, and valor were celebrated. Pure love was seen as incompatible with the temptations of the flesh; therefore, a distinction was made between love and sex, with sex having a lesser value. This distinction has been handed down through the ages and is still with us today.

Once again, what went on sexually with the people of the royal court during the Renaissance was very different from what occurred among the people of the streets and the fields. People outside the court were involved with music, drinking, dancing, and the theater. This was the age and time of Shakespeare.

A new sexual apparatus making its appearance at this time was something called a chastity belt. These belts allowed husbands to lock up their wives' genitals, just like they protected their money. They were designed to protect their wives from being raped. Thus, the belts were worn for their own good and safety, or so the story goes. It also made having an extramarital affair rather difficult.

Sex with one's marriage partner was mostly for the purpose of procreating, usually for an heir. Traditionally, it was not seen as something to be enjoyed, and respectable women were expected to lie passively during coitus. However, by the 15th century, there were contrary opinions. The biblical text of St. Paul, to "let the husband render to his wife what is due to her and likewise the wife to her husband," was often interpreted to mean that both sexes should experience satisfaction. There was also widespread acceptance of the theories of the ancient Greek physician, Galen, who taught that a woman who experienced orgasm was more likely to conceive a child, and husbands were therefore encouraged to help their wives achieve a climax. It therefore seems likely that despite the official teachings of the Church, many married couples enjoyed a fulfilling sexual relationship.

The Puritans

The Puritans were a group of people who grew discontented in the Church of England and worked toward religious, moral, and societal reforms. The writings and ideas of John Calvin, a leader in the Reformation, gave rise to Protestantism. Calvin's teachings were pivotal to the Christian revolt. Protestants contended that the Church of England had become a product of political struggles and man-made doctrines. The Puritans were one branch of dissenters who decided that the Church of England was beyond reform. Escaping persecution from Church leadership and the king, they came to America.(2)

The Puritans came across the Atlantic in search of a new home, at first in Jamestown in Virginia. The settlement was short-lived, and the next group of Puritans sailed to Plymouth, Massachusetts. Upon reaching land, they were weakened by their journey. As many as two or three people died each day during their first two months on land. Only 52 people survived that first year in Plymouth.

The most common belief about the Puritans and Pilgrims is that they were somehow against sex. The truth is that they did condemn playing cards, the theater, fancy clothes, and other things they believed were lures of the devil, but the Puritans were surprisingly open and frank about sex. They saw sex as a natural and joyous part of marriage that was to be plainly discussed and freely accepted.

If you look at the Puritans' circumstances when they first got to the New World, they needed to be sexually active from a reproductive point of view. When they landed on the beaches of this New World and they looked to the west, what did they see, other than a lot of trees? They saw thousands of Native Americans. They saw the tribes of the Iroquois Nation. They must have felt rather small in numbers and realized that if they were going to create a stronghold in this world, they would have to increase their population. Sex was great; they just had to make sure that it occurred within the context of marital relationship.

The Puritan sexual ethic, although severe and uncompromising, was primarily concerned with regulating the behavior that threatened the stability of the family. This was the beginning of what we call today "family values." The Puritans were concerned with and unforgiving of adultery and the birth of illegitimate children. Sexual activity within marriage was not strictly regulated. The Puritans were thus not against sex in principle, but rather were opposed to sexual behavior outside the bonds of marriage; i.e., what they believed to have been ordained by God and society.

The Puritans believed that man was by nature weak and therefore in need of constant self-examination, unremitting self-discipline, and hard work. The way to beat the devil and all his temptations was to stay busy working. Phrases such as "Keep your nose to the grindstone" and "Idle hands are the devil's workshop" translate into "If you keep your focus on work, you will steer clear of the devil's temptation." It can be argued that the Puritan work ethic has influenced how America was built; it continues to drive our current work culture.

The Victorian Period

The Victorian age marked the next historical turning point in sexual thinking. It roughly began with the reign of Queen Victoria in England beginning in 1837 and finished around the end of the 19th century. In previous periods, sexuality was always influenced by Christian religious beliefs. During the Victorian period, sexual attitudes were backed by the newly evolving science community, especially the field of medicine, which influenced sexual beliefs.

The overall Victorian attitude was that sex should be repressed and harnessed for what were considered more "character-building" pursuits. Where the Puritans were content to restrict sexual behavior to marriage, Victorians attempted to restrict sexual behavior within marriage as well. The whole society was focused on sexual repression. The essential Victorian philosophy was that sexual activity is primarily a procreation function and that those beyond their reproductive years should practice self-denial.

One of the more bizarre medical concepts that affected sexual behavior of the Victorian period revolved around a theory in which semen was viewed as a vital substance and its spillage a grievous and potentially lethal waste. The Victorians blamed all types of medical problems on the loss of semen. These included such diseases as leprosy, cancer and kidney disease. Headaches, blindness, epilepsy, loss of memory, digestive issues, impotency, tuberculosis, insanity, and even death were attributed to the loss of semen.

During the Victorian period, the repression of masturbation was a major obsession. The Victorians wanted to control the wasteful loss of semen because of the harmful possibilities. This is an example of the beliefs of the time. In her 1870 book, *A Solemn Appeal*, Ellen G. White writes: "If the practice [self-indulgence] is continued from the age of fifteen and upward, nature will protest against the abuse he has suffered, and continues to suffer, and will make them pay the penalty for the transgression of his laws, especially from the ages of thirty to forty-five, by numerous pains in the system, and various diseases, such as affection of the liver and lungs, neuralgia, rheumatism, affection of the spine, diseased kidneys, and cancerous tumors. Some of nature's fine machinery gives way, leaving a heavier task for the remaining to perform, which disorders nature's fine arrangement, and there is often a sudden breaking down of the constitution; and death is the result."(3)

The Victorian era is where so many of our myths about masturbation originated. One of the more common beliefs of the time was that masturbation would lead to blindness; a boy might get hairy palms. It was thought that masturbation could cause mental issues, sexual perversion, and reduce sexual functioning. Some of these myths are still passed on and circulating among young adolescents.

During the Victorian time frame, women were denied any sexual experience, except what was required to produce a child. Women had to dress in a way to keep any exposure of the flesh hidden. They wore clothing, including corsets and hoops, that blocked any ability to be near their actual bodies. They wore these dresses, despite their actual living conditions. Just think of how women dressed during the development of the American West. They walked around in those dresses even if it was 100 degrees outside.

The Victorian wife's "duty" was to serve her husband and family. This was her sole focus, protecting the sanctity of her family. She had sex just to please her husband, fulfill his needs, and give him children. During the Victorian era, economics regarding marriage was put ahead of romance. Many arranged marriages were made more as a business deal than because of romance or love.

Another way in which the Victorians tried to repress sexuality was through the use of language. They would not use words that had any anatomical link. You wouldn't want to say at the dinner table, "Could you pass the turkey breast?" or "Could I have a chicken leg?"

During this time, the Victorians used all kinds of euphemisms for anything with a sexual reference. One of the first books that I read about sex was called *Memoirs of a Woman of Pleasure (*popularly known as *Fanny Hill*). This is an erotic novel by John Cleveland, first published in England in 1748. This novel is considered "the first original English prose pornography, and the first pornography to use the form of the novel."(4) One of the most prosecuted and banned books in history, it has become a synonym for obscenity. When I read this book at the young age of 12, I couldn't understand what was being talked about because of all the euphemisms, but somehow I knew it was about sex.

During this period, sexual activity was repressed by Victorian society in general, but when sexual expression is shut down, people find a way to get their needs met. During this time, men discovered a way to get their sexual needs met, even if their wives were not available to them. What the sexual repression of this time did was to create an incredible sexual underground. Red-light districts appeared where prostitution was rampant in every major European city, as well as the major cities of America.

In her article, *Fallen Woman*, Amy Greene says, "There were many prostitutes during the Victorian era. Most were lower-class women, with the exception of the mistresses kept by upper-class men. According to Victorian standards, respectable women did not consider sexual intercourse pleasurable. It was their duty to be intimate with their husbands. Having affairs was disgraceful (Waters). Prostitutes, on the other hand, were sexually intimate with men because they enjoyed sex. Men enjoyed prostitutes because they could not enjoy their wives. Victorian femininity was not defined by sexual pleasure, while Victorian masculinity was defined by sexual pleasure and conquest.

"Prostitutes did not necessarily 'enjoy' their sexual encounters with men, as Victorians tended to believe. Prostitution was their survival. Lower-class women did not become prostitutes because they wanted to. They became prostitutes because they had no alternate choice for survival. There were few options that allowed women to live off her own income instead of her family's, and once she entered the profession, Victorian society did not allow her back into 'respectable' society."(5)

The philosophical end of the Victorian period was brought down by one individual, Dr. Sigmund Freud. Dr. Freud was a well-respected doctor and scientist in Vienna, Austria. He was held in high esteem by the European medical community, which gave him a lot of influence on the thinking of the time. Freud's beliefs attacked one of the basic sexual theoretical underpinnings of the

Victorian era: that all sexual repression leads to mental neuroses. This belief was in complete opposition to Victorian sexual thinking.

The Roaring Twenties

After the end of World War I, Americans wanted to get back to a normal life and have a good time. In 1917, Congress passed the National Prohibition Act, known informally as the Volstead Act, to carry out the intent of the Eighteenth Amendment, which established prohibition against alcohol in the United States. Just imagine all these soldiers coming back from a very ugly war and being told by the government that they couldn't consume alcohol, at least legally.

Just as the Victorians' efforts to repress sex in society other than for reproduction had the result of creating a very sexually active underground, a similar backlash occurred with the government's prohibition of alcohol. An illegal underground of the consumption, distribution, and manufacturing of alcohol evolved.

When Americans are told they can't do something behaviorally or socially, they tend to want to do it more, and this is what occurred during the 1920s in terms of alcohol consumption. So, from an underground point of view, alcohol became the drug of choice that fueled the social party attitude that was the Roaring Twenties.

Socially, sex was expressed in many different ways during this time, which was in complete contrast with the previous Victorian period. Sexuality was expressed through the popular music of the time. Jazz and dancing were a major part of the party scene that would occur in the "speakeasies" and nightclubs in major American cities.

Everything changed in the Roaring Twenties. Sex in the 1920s was revolutionized with the widespread use of the motorcar, as well as seeing the steaming actors and actresses of the silver screen. With sex on everyone's mind, it's not surprising that many books would be sold to a populace obsessed with sex. Like many aspects of the 1920s, the best-selling novel was a new invention of the time.

The "sex novel," as it became known, reflected the shifting moralities of the decade. With the emergence of the femme fatale, feminine sexuality came into its own. Critics and moral pundits screamed from every rooftop about the loosening morals of American society, while the "immoral" writings of D. H. Lawrence flew off the shelves.(6) It was during the 1920s that the term flapper made its appearance. A flapper was a young woman who sought out pleasure for pleasure's sake and freedom from the bondage of traditional conformity; the flapper became the independent modern woman.

During this time, the economy was booming. People were living the high life, due to the rise in the stock market. The only problem was that the general public was buying stock on margin. This meant that they were, in a sense, borrowing money to finance their stock purchases. It would be like buying Google stock today with a credit card. All the prosperity was built on an economic house of cards.

The stock market crashed, and the American economy collapsed on what was called Black Tuesday on October 29, 1929. It was the most devastating stock market crash in the history of the United States, taking into consideration the full extent and duration of its fallout. The crash signaled the beginning of the ten-year-long Great Depression that affected all Western industrialized countries. The Depression did not end in the United States until the onset of American mobilization for World War II at the end of 1941. (7)

The Great Depression and the 1930s

During economic hard times, people tend to become more conservative sexually. During the Great Depression of the 1930s, this was also the case. When people are out of work and have many children to feed and raise, they face a major financial challenge. The lack of effective birth control methods during this time put a damper on being sexually active. Women's fashions made a dramatic shift from the sexualized dress of the 1920s to the more sexually conservative 1930s.

When sexuality is repressed in society at large, it seems to give rise to violence. This pattern could be seen during the 1930s with the rise of celebrity bank robbers. Bank robbers such as Bonnie and Clyde, John Dillinger, Pretty Boy Floyd, and the Ma Barker gang were waging war against the banks of the Midwest. Criminals in some way provided a vicarious release of the working people's anger toward the banks that foreclosed on their farms and houses. There were even tales of how Pretty Boy Floyd gave some of the money he stole to farmers to pay off their mortgages. These stories are echoed in the lyrics of a Woody Guthrie song, *Pretty Boy Floyd*.

Hard times had another effect on people's personal lives. "Unemployment permitted a great deal more companionship between young men and young women, which ordinarily would have led to marriage. The only thing lacking was money. The arrangements called, simply, 'living together' became common. Often the man or woman was married, and couldn't get, couldn't afford, or didn't want a divorce. Sometimes the man simply refused to marry, and the woman took him into her home or moved into his as the next best thing." (8)

World War II

When Japan invaded Pearl Harbor in Hawaii on December 7, 1941, America entered World War II against Japan and Germany. With millions of men facing death at any moment, it is no real surprise that many sought release and escape in sex. When war comes, sexual attitudes shift from delayed gratification to an attitude of living for the moment, because who knows if you will even come back alive? With so many men in the armed forces, away from women, sexuality became a major focus. Hollywood pin-up pictures were seen wherever they could be displayed. Photos of Betty Grable, Rita Hayworth, Lana Turner, Veronica Lake, Susan Hayward, and many other Hollywood celebrities were on the list.

Dancing to big band music was another way for the soldiers to express their sexuality. It was a way for men and women to meet when so many men were away from their homes. Some of the Hollywood stars and sex symbols of the time would tour the various military bases overseas to help sexually entertain the troops.

With so many men fighting overseas, the women of America had to step in and take their places in the defense plants, working around the clock throughout the country. This was a major change in the roles women had played prior to the war. During World War II, there was a change in the image of women, but it was only superficial and temporary. The reality was that most women returned to being homemakers during the postwar prosperity of the 1950s. However, the road taken by women in the work force during World War II continued into the future. Society had changed. The daughters and granddaughters of the women who worked in the factories continued on the road blazed by their mothers and grandmothers.

World War II sparked changes in views about sex and love. It created a new wave of love connections, sexual encounters, hasty marriages, and prostitution, and helped generate the second wave of the women's movement.(9)

The 1950s and the Baby Boom Period

After the end of World War II, all the young men and women coming back wanted to settle down and return to what they called a normal life. They had put their early twenties on hold to fight in the war effort, so they had a great deal of pent-up desire. They wanted to get married and raise a family. They wanted to own a home and return to work. These attitudes gave rise to the biggest period of sexual reproduction in recorded history. It became known as the baby boom. The American federal government helped in this cause with the legislation of the GI Bill, which aided returning veterans by giving them the ability to buy homes and access to higher education through easy financing.

The 1950s were a period in which America built the suburbs of the major urban centers throughout the country. Reasonably priced housing allowed for extensive home building and demand. Everyone wanted their own home with two kids; they wanted what they thought was the pursuit of the American Dream.

The 1950s were a very sexual time, but sexual in a very conservative way. The sexual activity was all about reproduction—within the context of marriage. Everybody was expected to wait until they married before having sexual intercourse. For a woman, being a virgin was extremely important. The Madonna-whore dichotomy came back in a big way.

Even in the context of marriage, sex was rather conservative. Married people slept in twin beds. No one talked about someone being pregnant. Instead, they would say a woman was in the family way. Basically, sex was for men and something the woman did for him, but if she were to become too sexually assertive, she would be judged. The children and the family were the main concerns for the wife. If her interest deviated from taking care of the family such as having a career or profession, she would be judged by her peers and family as being a narcissistic deviation—or just plain selfish.

If a man got a woman pregnant out of wedlock, then usually he was expected to do the right thing and marry the woman, even if he knew he didn't love her. Getting an abortion usually wasn't an option. If the woman wanted one, it was a nightmare of an experience. People who were rich probably bought off a doctor to perform an illegal procedure. If you didn't have the money, then it was done usually in some back alley, or you could go to Mexico, where it most likely was some haphazard medical procedure that could be physically dangerous. Many couples got married because they had to, due to a pending pregnancy, not because they wanted to. This fact might have had an influence on why so many couples got divorced in the late 1960s.

Even though the 1950s and early 1960s were generally seen as a conservative sexual period, sexual changes were occurring in society at large. "Sexual attitudes during the 1950s were in a state of transition. On one hand, as Albert Ellis writes in *The American Sexual Tragedy* (1954), a woman was obliged 'to make herself infinitely sexually desirable—but finally approachable only in legal marriage.' But men were encouraged to adopt the swinging bachelor's lifestyle represented by *Playboy* magazine, which debuted in 1953. The magazine's notorious pictorials of naked women, *Playboy* publisher Hugh Hefner explained, were symbols 'of disobedience, a triumph of sexuality, an end of Puritanism.' Hefner's announcement of the death of puritanism might have been a bit premature—the sexual revolution was still a decade away—but sexual values were clearly changing. And perhaps, as such scientific studies as the one conducted by Alfred Kinsey and associates seem to suggest, Americans were never particularly puritanical."(10)

Another expression of sexuality during this time was the birth and popularity of rock-and-roll music, especially among American youth. The name of this type of music was really an African American euphemism for having sex. Rock music allowed young people the ability to move and dance and set their bodies free. It was all about being sexual, which is why many parents at the time hated this music. It gave young people an avenue to express themselves in such a way as to break out of the anti-sex pressure of the time.

Although rock and roll was mostly part of black culture in the early 1950s, it soon transitioned to white youth, brought on by the popularity of Elvis Presley. He represented a certain sexuality that threatened the conservative established society. The way he would shake his hips when he performed made many people uncomfortable. When Presley appeared on national television, they cut the camera angle so you couldn't see his hips. Certain religious groups believed that rock-and-roll music represented the "devil's music" and should be banned.

In the 1950s, sex was something that you saved for marriage. If a woman was sexually active outside the context of marriage, she was seen as "easy" and judged as being virtually a prostitute. Of course, men who were sexually active outside of marriage were just seen as playboys. So the double standard for sexual behavior was still going strong during this time.

The Sexual Revolution of the 1960s

The sexual revolution, also known as the time of sexual liberation, marked a time that involved the rejection of typical gender roles. It was a social movement that challenged what individuals had previously seen as sexual norms. Acceptance of intercourse outside of monogamous, heterosexual, marriages increased, which gave individuals more freedom, as well as a feeling of being less deviant. New contraceptives hit the market. The availability of the birth control pill in particular gave women the power and control they never had before in this way (Crooks, 2011). In the 1960s, intrauterine devices (IUDs) were first manufactured and marketed in the United States; these gave women even more options in terms of birth control methods (Kathleen, 2011).(11)

"For all these sexual changes both socially and technologically some sociologists and historians argue that there wasn't really a revolution in the true sense of what a revolution truly means. These changes to sexual attitudes and behaviors during the period are often today referred to generally under the blanket metaphor of sexual revolution.

"Whilst the term revolution implies radical and widespread change, this was not necessarily the case. Even in the liberal sixties, conservative, traditionalist views were widely held. Using the term revolution may be too much of an overstatement."(12)

The real change was the advent and popular use of the birth control pill. This pharmaceutical invention had a profound effect on people's sexual behavior and attitudes. With the birth control pill, women now had the ability to free themselves from the fear of getting pregnant from the act of sexual intercourse. In the 1960s, having a large family wasn't seen as an asset. The pill gave couples the ability to limit the number of children they had, while at the same time not limiting their sex life. Smaller families gave couples greater mobility to travel, which was important to major corporations so they could move their employees and executives around the country, increasing their economic possibilities.

There was a type of backlash to the birth control pill, which, on one hand, offered protection from pregnancy, but on the other had the effect of pressuring women into having more intercourse. With the pill, women didn't seem to have an excuse to say no, unless they had some type of sexually transmitted disease. It seems as if the pill took away the serious aspects of sexual intercourse, so it became "hip" to engage in it a lot more often.

Some of the sexual social significance of this period was that sex became a major focal point of the culture through media and advertising. Sex was being used to sell everything. Also, there was an increased emphasis on sex and personal relations as the basic source of happiness in people's lives. All the commercialization and trivialization of sex made advances into people's private lives, which took away the deeper meaning of intimacy and love as being essential elements to a fulfilling sexual experience.

"Sex, love, and rock and roll" was one of the popular slogans of the 1960s. This was how many of the youth of the time lived their lives. One could say that the sexual revolution of the 1960s was a backlash against the conservative, repressive 1950s. The baby boom generation became the "Woodstock Nation" that went sexually crazy, skinny-dipping in the park totally "stoned out" on marijuana and LSD. I personally went to San Francisco looking for "free love" with the "hippie chicks," but didn't find any. I wasn't alone in this pursuit.

The 1960s were a very polarized time within American culture and society. There were the "straights" and the "freaks," with the straights being part of what was called "the Establishment"—those who conformed to the values of the status quo of the time, which included materialism, capitalism, the pursuit of the American Dream, and supporting the war in Vietnam. The freaks, on the other hand, were the long-haired hippies, the student demonstrators against the war effort, and all of those people who were antiestablishment.

The youth culture of the time was very sexually and sensuously expressive. All the senses were stimulated whenever the freaks were together, either in mass gatherings or in private homes. The motivation of sensuality probably was highly influenced by the use of psychedelic drugs, especially LSD. People dressed in bright colors and in tie-dyed patterns. Hippies wanted a way to escape from the strict social norm of the 1950s, and the new tie-dye fashion was just one way of expressing their free-spirited nature.(13) Visual stimulation was very much a part of this period. When you went to listen to rock music, you didn't just listen to music, you were treated to what was called a psychedelic light show that accompanied the music.

Besides the visual stimulation, smells were always present at any gathering. Some of the odors were used to mask the smell of marijuana and/or body odor, but they were pretty strong. The use of incense burning, fragrant candles, and the smell of one particular fragrance called patchouli oil was common. This was all happening before we ever heard the term aromatherapy.

During this era, another sense that was very prolific was touch. Public displays of hugging and holding were commonplace. There were no more worries about public displays of affection that had been such concerns of the previous generation. The idea of giving and receiving massages became very popular.

Sound was best represented during this time by the pervasive presence of music everywhere. The music of the time was the soundtrack to people's lives as events and experiences occurred. Music was the common denominator. It wasn't just rock music; people listened to different types of music such as jazz and the Indian sitar music of Ravi Shankar. The type of music you listened to was something that identified you as being different from the straights.

All of these sensual elements played a role in affecting the way people made love at this time. I think these sensual elements still have an influence today, if only with a minority of people who still remember the 1960s.

"The sexual revolution of the 1960's is an era unimaginable to many of today's young people. Granted, many teenagers and twenty-something adults engage in risky sexual acts and adopt a freethinking view towards sex. However, the greater part of the population cannot, and will never fully comprehend the concept of sex and freedom. This perception was born in the sixties, and has transcended the way Americans view their bodies and their sexuality.

"The sexual behavior of Americans changed within one decade. Before the 1960's American youths had somewhat of a protected view of sexuality. Prior to this decade, many journalist[s] and psychologist[s] wrote articles and commentary speaking of sexual freedom. These writing[s] made outspoken claims such as 10% of the American population was gay, and that most Americans masturbated. These taboo topics were rarely spoken among the masses. Most journalists during the late 1950's and early 1960's were encouraging sexual freedom. Older ones were less apt to embrace such a liberal view towards sexuality, however, the younger generation quickly jumped on the sexual revolution bandwagon.

"Women began to take control of their sexuality and trade in long skirts for short minis without pantyhose. Moreover, revealing necklines became the custom, and bras were discarded as a mark of independence.

"Of course, the sexual revolution of the 1960's encompassed more than provocative clothing. Homosexuals who lived in secret came out of the closet, and casual sex was on the rise. It was typical to stumble upon two people having sex in a public place.

"The sexual revolution of the 1960's gave the American population the free will to live their life without feeling ashamed."(14)

The 1970s: The Changing Morality

The so-called sexual revolution continued after the 1960s, and was considered by many to be the most shocking social trend in the 1970s. This revolution, an outgrowth of the counterculture, cast aside traditional sexual restraints and began a decade of alternative eroticism, experimentation, and promiscuity. This was facilitated in part by the development of the birth control pill and other contraceptives.

Americans in the 1970s broke many sexual taboos. Interracial dating, open homosexuality, communal living, casual nudity, and dirty language all seemed to indicate a profound change in sexual behavior. Sexual activity among the young especially increased. Surveys during the 1970s reported that by age 19, four-fifths of all males and two-thirds of all females had engaged in sex. Fashion designers promoted a new sensuality, producing miniskirts, hot pants, halter tops, and form-fitting clothes designed to accentuate women's sexuality.(15)

The 1970s seemed like one big sexual party, especially the second half of the decade. The party was fueled by a new drug of choice: cocaine. In the previous decade, marijuana was so prevalent, but now there was a white powder that seemed to be everywhere. The common myth at the time was that it couldn't hurt you and wasn't addictive. The destruction to people's lives that this myth created became abundantly clear within a few years.

"Individuals turned their attention to this high-energy producing and glamorous drug that represented the perfect companion to the disco culture that exploded in the mid-1970s. Cocaine use spread extremely quickly throughout America at the end of the 1970s, gaining popularity not just in discos nationwide, but also among various classes and types of individuals hoping to attain its pleasurable and energy-producing effects. The popularity of cocaine can be partially attributed to widespread ignorance of its harmful side effects, which in turn established it as somewhat of a socially accepted drug."(16)

Sexual promiscuity was commonplace. The idea of being married seemed restrictive and wasn't where the fun and excitement existed. People wanted to "do their own thing," and the singles lifestyle seemed very attractive. Married couples experimented with alternatives to the institution of marriage with the concept of "open marriage." A couple could have a sexual relationship with someone outside their marriage, as long everything was done with their spouse's consent. Some couples experimented with wife swapping and becoming swingers. You might say they were trying to have their cake and eat it too, but I think for most, this experiment ended in disaster to their marriage.

The 1980s and the Age of HIV

At the beginning of the 1980s, the Moral Majority, a conservative movement, came to the national forefront, led by the Reverend Jerry Falwell. Falwell represented the rise of the religious right, and their reaction to the sexual revolution and all the changes that were occurring that they found immoral. In general, the negative consequences of the freewheeling sexuality of the 1960s and 1970s were catching up with the population at large. The psychological community became concerned about the issues created for the children of divorced parents. Feminist critiques of the objectification of women in the rise of pornography became more vocal.

Given all the media exposure regarding the concerns about the impact of the sexual revolution, people's behavior in the beginning of the 1980s didn't really change and become more conservative. Maybe some young people were waiting for marriage before they had sex or used condoms, but high school sexuality was very active. Girls were losing their virginity without the guilt of previous generations. Losing one's virginity became no big deal; it was seen as being "normal." Porn theaters went out of business due to the affordability of the VCR machine. Now people could go to their local video store and rent X-rated adult video material and watch in the privacy of their own homes. Pornography was moving into the mainstream of the culture and was becoming big business.

With the widespread use of cocaine in the 1970s, people began to see that this was a highly addictive drug by the following decade. During the 1980s, a new form of cocaine was hitting the streets in the form of crack—a cheaper, smokable, and more potent version of powdered cocaine. Crack addiction became an epidemic in the 1980s and brought widespread destruction to people's lives, as they would become easily addicted to the drug.

The most significant event of the 1980s to impact people's sex lives was the discovery and subsequent pandemic known as HIV/AIDS (human immunodeficiency virus infection/acquired immunodeficiency syndrome). Sometime in the mid-1980s, gay men began dying in large numbers from a disease called AIDS. Not much was known as to what caused this disease, and there was no known cure at the time.

The public became terrified as it became clear that the disease could be contracted by heterosexuals as well. At first, there was great fear as to how the disease could be contracted. Could you get it from kissing someone, holding their hand, or from drinking from a glass that someone else used? Later, it became clear that it was contracted through sexual relations with someone who was HIV-positive. Another way to get AIDS was through sharing intravenous drugs, using contaminated needles, or by way of blood transfusions.

The effect of the AIDS epidemic was to change the way people lived their sexual lives. There was a lot more fear of STDs—AIDS being the scariest of all—but people were much more anxious about lesser threats like herpes, so there was a big "safe-sex" campaign. Caution about carefree do-whatever-feels-good sexuality wasn't just coming from conservatism, but from a lot of different sources.

The idea of being sexually involved with someone you didn't really know or have an established relationship with became a threat to your life. Before, if you got an STD, you could get a penicillin shot and you were good to go. Now, the idea of being single didn't have the same appeal as it did previously. The old values of commitment, monogamy, and marriage had a greater appeal from a sexual point of view. By the end of the 1980s, the sexually free lifestyle had changed.

Sex in the 1990s

During the 1990s, sexual behavior in America became much more conservative and restrained in comparison to the previous two decades. The reason for this was that the AIDS/HIV epidemic had taken a strong hold in influencing people's sexual choices. The term safe sex became a part of the sexual vocabulary. The media proliferation of the concept put the fear of HIV on everyone's consciousness.

Children in middle and high school were losing their innocence through sex education about safe-sex methods. They were being taught how to use condoms, not for protection as a birth control method, but more as a way to prevent the spread of the HIV virus. Even though some religious groups protested and tried to block this type of sex education, the fear of HIV prevailed.

Even with the campaign to enlighten the youth of the time, how much safe sex was actually practiced might be a different reality. The belief of teenagers in their immortality and their own sense of denial may have gotten in the way of the actual practice of safe sex. Among adults, the practice of safe sex meant monogamy was the way to protect yourself against HIV. Even though the risk was high, people didn't always stay sexually committed and many times exposed their partners to health risks.

During the 1990s, a new drug came on the scene, especially popular with those in their twenties. It was called Ecstasy, or MDMA, which is a synthetic substance, usually sold in a pill form. It was developed as medication to help psychotherapy patients dealing with self-examination and to improve intimate communication. It became known as the "love drug" by some because many people who used it experienced a sense of empathy and connection with others while they were under its influence. By the 1990s, it became a standard part of rave parties, which were all-night dance parties.

"The dynamic of homosexual politics in the 1990s consisted of gays and lesbians trying to establish themselves in mainstream American life and the efforts of conservatives to resist such a fundamental cultural change. Many Americans, meanwhile, seem to have drifted toward a somewhat uneasy accommodation with homosexuality."(17)

Gay rights was a prominent topic in the United States in the 1990s. During the Clinton administration, the issue of homosexual rights in the American military came to the forefront. Whether or not homosexuals should be discharged if they were openly gay became the topic of the time. "Known as 'don't ask, don't tell,' the policy was presented as a way to allow gays in the military to serve without fear of discharge or other penalty as long as they did not reveal their sexual orientation, but it did not significantly change the precarious status of gay soldiers."(18)

Another front in the gay rights movement surfacing in the 1990s was the political fight for same-sex marriage, to give homosexual couples the same legal rights as traditional heterosexual married couples. Congress reacted to this movement with the passing of the Defense of Marriage Act in 1996, restricting the federal definition of marriage to heterosexual couples and denying certain benefits, such as filing joint tax returns, to legally married same-sex couples; the act has been challenged in the courts. The Supreme Court of the United States struck down the Defense of Marriage Act in June 2013 on the basis that it is unconstitutional.

The New Millennium and Beyond

As for the trends and changes since 2000, it's hard to tell. You decide from your perspective. Not enough time has passed to give enough distance to see clearly, in my view. One thing that is clear is that people's behavior and attitudes toward the subject of human sexuality will continue to evolve and change. Whether these changes are good or bad depends on a person's value system. It will be interesting to see the impact of the digital age and the influence of the Internet on people's sexuality in the future.

Works Cited

1. http://www.oddee.com/item_96646.aspx#2W6lLfZSIuc9h74I.99
2. www.ux1.eiu.edu/~cfrnb/puritans.html
3. White, Ellen G. *A Solemn Appeal*. 1870, copyright 2010, Ellen G. White Estate, Inc.
4. http://en.wikipedia.org/wiki/Fanny_Hill#cite_note-3
5. http://cai.ucdavis.edu/waters-sites/prostitution/FallenWomen.htm)
6. http://www.1920s-fashion-and-music.com/1920s-sex.html#ixzz2TOtjGKh0
7. http://en.wikipedia.org/wiki/Wall_Street_Crash_of_1929
8. http://www.oldmagazinearticles.com/1930s-Sex Coronet Magazine, 1947
9. http://www.philadelphiaweekly.com/events/On-the-Home-Front-and-Beyond-Love—Sex-During-World-War-II-189073121.html
10. http://www.bookrags.com/history/america-1950s-lifestyles-and-social-trends/sub8.html
11. http://historyofsexuality.umwblogs.org/
12. http://en.wikipedia.org/wiki/Sexual_revolution_in_1960s_United_States#cite_note-2
13. http://iml.jou.ufl.edu/projects/Spring09/blake_e/history.html
14. http://www.loti.com/sexual_revolution.htm The Sexual Revolution by Valencia Higuera.
15. http://my-retrospace.blogspot.com/2009/12/sexual-revolution.html
16. American Studies Seminar at the College of William and Mary in the fall of 2007.
17. http://www.bookrags.com/history/america-1990s-lifestyles-and-social-trends/sub14.html

18. http://www.infoplease.com/encyclopedia/society/gay-rights-movement.html#ixzz2X51ur2LL

2

Sexual Socialization and Sex Education

Now that I have presented a historical perspective on the development of human sexuality through the ages of Western civilization up to the new millennium, I want to take a sociological approach as to how the past becomes part of an individual's sexual experience. Most individuals are socialized sexually through the major sociological institutions in our culture. Sometimes, this sociological process is done quite deliberately and consciously, whereas in other situations, it occurs on very subtle levels of conscious awareness.

The key pragmatic point in understanding the sexual socialization process is that once a person knows how they were socialized, they can make attitudinal or behavioral changes if they are so inclined. We don't have to be victims of our past. We can make changes today to liberate ourselves from the different institutions with which we came in contact while we were growing up.

Parents and Our Families

The first sociological institution that begins our sexual socialization process is our parents and family of origin. Our parents have a great deal of impact in shaping our sexual attitudes because they get to us first before any other influences. As children, we give what our parents say a tremendous amount of power because to children, our parents are all-knowing and the experts on any subject, including the subject of sex.

The problem is that parents are not experts on the subject of human sexuality and generally are not that comfortable discussing the subject. This discomfort with the subject matter is compounded by the fact that many people in American culture believe that sex education should occur in the home. This social expectation puts added pressure on parents to carry the psychological weight in educating their children about sex.

Even the most sophisticated, highly educated parents may feel paralyzed by not knowing what to tell their children about sex and at what age to have the discussions. As a result, they wait for their children's questions to arise regarding a particular topic. That's assuming that their children ask anything at all. All this uncertainty about when and what to discuss creates an atmosphere of discomfort for both the parents and their children, and as a result, the topic of sex is often avoided or just given a cursory approach.

When I ask students or patients about how sex was talked about in their homes growing up, they often say that their parents didn't even discuss the topic. What psychological message does this send to our children? If they know the topic exists, but isn't discussed, what does that tell children on a nonverbal level? It tells them that there is something wrong or negative about the subject of sex. Consequently, early on in our sexual development, we may get the message that there is something negative about sex, mainly because of the silence surrounding the topic.

Recently, I have heard stories of parents who don't fit this stereotype. These parents want to be completely open and tell their children all about what they know regarding sex. They want to convey a healthy and open atmosphere to their children regarding the subject of sex, to break the trend that was passed down by their parents. This sounds good, but might be overwhelming to a child, unless the parents have a good sense of timing.

When I give public seminars, parents often ask what they should tell their children about sex, and when. The answer is that there isn't really a specific time because all children mature and develop at different rates. So, the answer is when it makes sense for your child, and only that parent knows when the time is right. I do know that children's age of innocence regarding certain aspects of sex has gotten younger and younger in the past 40 years, especially with the HIV epidemic, the proliferation of sex on the Internet, and education regarding the prevention of sexual abuse.

Probably the real sex education that occurs in the home is not so much what is verbally expressed by a child's parents, but more unconsciously by what children witness every day living with their parents. The behavioral interactions between parents have a greater impact than what they say. How much affection occurs between the parents, their attitude about nudity, whether the parents flirt with each, whether they make time for each other away from their children—these all play a role in a child's sexual education.

Children absorb the general emotional atmosphere of their parents' relationship like a sponge. They are generally unconscious of their experience, but it's their take-away from their childhood that plays a role in their own adult relationships. Were their parents cold and distant from each other? Where they just staying together until their children graduated high school before seeking a divorce? Children pick up on the general atmosphere of their home, which can affect their relationships later in life.

If parents want to educate their children, they must be comfortable with the subject of sex. It's not the information that the parents give their children in the moment that they will remember, but the emotional atmosphere in which the information is delivered. I don't remember so much what my mother told me about where babies came from, but how emotionally uptight she was when she gave me the lecture. When she said, "We have to have a talk," I thought I was in trouble and was going to be punished. I tell parents that if they aren't comfortable talking to their kids about sex, it's better that they find some resources where the children can get helpful sex information without the stressful environment.

When sex education does occur in the home, the discussion is usually the responsibility of the mother. She is often the one to initiate the talk with her children. Generally, the information is limited to the subjects of menstruation and pregnancy. "According to interviews conducted for the Kaiser Family Foundation in 2000, 65% of parents believe that sex education should encourage young people to delay sexual activity but also prepare them to use birth control and practice safe sex once they do become sexually active, In fact, public opinion is overwhelmingly supportive of sexuality education that goes beyond abstinence. Moreover, public opinion polls over the years have routinely shown that the vast majority of Americans favor broader sex education programs over those that teach only abstinence."(1)

What do you remember your parents telling you about sex? Many parents give their children one-line injunctions like "Be safe and put a raincoat on it," "Save it until you meet that special person," or "Don't get her pregnant." These parental sexual messages may have been all that some people received from their parents regarding sex education in the home.

Sex education from our parents usually falls short of preparing children for adult relationships. I don't really blame parents because they do the best they can, given their own limitations from their childhood experiences with their own parents.

Organized Religion

Invariably, my early discussions with couples and individuals in therapy come around to the subject of how their religious beliefs had an impact on their sexuality. Depending on the religious persuasion of their parents, children get different sexual messages. The messages and information that come from religious organizations are slanted to their own belief systems, and as a result, the objectivity of the organization is questionable.

Some religions are very direct about specific sexual dos and don'ts. Other times, the sexual messages are indirect and left to individual interpretation. This creates problems because a young person with very little knowledge or experience about sex is unable to check out their interpretations with reality. As a consequence, many false assumptions and myths have developed around sex. These beliefs stay with us into adulthood, negatively affecting our sexual behavior.

Generally, a child's religious affiliation has the greatest impact on shaping their sexual attitudes when they are young adolescents. When a child is moving into puberty, their sexual hormones are making themselves known by creating secondary sex characteristics. These changes create a large amount of sexual curiosity and quest for sexual knowledge. So, whatever messages their religion directs their way, it has full impact because of the child's thirst for sexual knowledge.

What I find in the adults I work with in therapy is that the sexual messages and attitudes instilled by their religion are still a part of their present-day thinking—even if they no longer believe or identify with the religion they followed during their adolescence. I find this to be more the case with conservative or orthodox religions because they give stronger and clearer sexual messages and beliefs.

For example, it's common for a child who was raised as a Roman Catholic and was exposed to the sexual teachings of the Church during their adolescence to still have these beliefs affect them psychologically in adult life. This is true even with adults who say that they no longer go to church and have distanced themselves from some of the basic Church principles. They still experience sexual guilt if their sexual behavior conflicts with the Church's teachings. This conflict also occurs with people who were raised with other religious denominations.

One of the more common beliefs or teachings of most Christian denominations is that sex should occur within the bonds of marriage. Premarital sex is generally regarded as a sin. This belief creates a problem for people who buy into the concept of controlling and repressing sex outside the context of a marital relationship. They're damned if they do, and damned if they don't.

Those who are damned if they don't are the many women I see who put their sexuality on hold until the right man comes along for them to marry. They may wait for years. Then, once they are married, suddenly it's okay to be sexual and they are expected to turn their sexual feelings on, as if they were wired to a light switch. Fortunately, human beings aren't put together like electronic devices. Most of us find it virtually impossible to suddenly respond sexually when we've been repressing such feelings for a long time. Even though we suddenly have permission to be sexual, the old "you shouldn't" tapes are still grinding away in the background. As a result, we feel guilty, which gets in the way of enjoying this area of the human experience.

This double bind can apply equally to women and men. Usually, we receive the double message that it's not really okay to be sexual before marriage, but for young men, well, "boys will be boys." You might assume that the incidence of teenage sex argues that the taboo against premarital sex has disappeared, and compared to the past, this is true. The influence of this belief depends on how strongly the individual adheres to their religious beliefs.

The Public Education System

Traditionally, in public schools before the 1980s and the age of HIV/AIDS, adolescents were rarely given any information on sexual matters because discussion of these issues was considered taboo. Such instruction was traditionally left to a child's parents, and often this was put off until just before a child's marriage. As previously discussed, it is clear that many parents aren't equipped to teach their children about sex. This deficiency became increasingly evident by the increasing incidence of teen pregnancies, especially in Western countries after the 1960s. In an effort to reduce such pregnancies, sex education programs were instituted, initially over strong opposition from parent and religious groups. In the 1980s, school systems were forced to increase their efforts at sex education due to the concerns of the HIV epidemic and other sexually transmitted diseases, as well as concerns about sexual assault and abuse. Even though the schools make efforts to inform their students about current sexual issues, they continue to run into the conservative religious organizations that try to block these efforts. I can remember in the 1960s in Orange County in Southern California there were groups that thought sex education in the schools was a Communist political plot against our country.

Today, many parents look to the schools to provide sex education to their children because of their own discomfort with the subject. Other parents are bitterly opposed to sex education in the schools for a variety of reasons and still believe it's the responsibility of the parents to educate their children about sex. In this difficult political environment, sex education in public schools has come a long way over the past 40 years, but it still falls short of what is really needed. Living in fear of community pressure groups, the schools try their best to present needed information. Not everyone's school sex education experience is the same, especially for those who went to private religious schools. The experience varies from what part of the country a person went to school and their age. This is something I have experienced myself and have heard from the many students who have told me their experience of sex education in the California public schools.

Historically, sex education in public schools has primarily emphasized biology and reproduction. The first sex education in school that I remember was in the sixth grade. The boys got to go out and play on the playground and the girls went into the auditorium to watch a movie. It's not that we minded having extra time on the playground, but we thought it strange that we didn't get to see the movie that the girls were watching. Somehow, we knew that it had something to do with sex (whatever that meant to us at the time), but didn't know what aspect. We made jokes and laughed about it, but that was about it. Later, I found out that it was a film about menstruation. Apparently, they thought the boys weren't mature enough to handle the film or didn't need to know about the subject of menstruation.

My next sex education experience was in middle school, around seventh or eighth grade. This experience occurred during my gym class and only included boys. For a week of school, we didn't have to suit up for gym, and instead, we went into a regular classroom with my gym coach as the teacher. I didn't mind not suiting up for gym, something I didn't like too much at that time, but I thought it was strange having my gym coach as a teacher.

Gym teachers at that time were males who acted like they were Marine drill sergeants. They had crew cuts and wore skinny black ties with short-sleeved white shirts and called us men. They were very intimidating in their demeanor to young 13-year-old adolescents. For me, it wasn't so much about the content of what the gym coach said, but the surrounding emotional experience that had the most long-lasting impact on my sexual history.

On the first day of class, the gym teacher started talking to us about the evils of drugs. I knew nothing about drugs at this time. It was 1963 and we were all very innocent about such topics. We saw films such as *Reefer Madness* (originally released as *Tell Your Children* and sometimes titled as *The Burning Question*, *Dope Addict*, *Doped Youth*, and *Love Madness*), a 1936 American propaganda exploitation film revolving around the melodramatic events that ensue when high school students are lured by pushers to try marijuana—from a hit-and-run accident, to manslaughter, suicide, attempted rape, and descent into madness. This was the school's attempt to scare us so we would never touch something called marijuana. The message was, if you try marijuana, you will be using heroin in no time. I don't think this attempt at preventing baby boomers from using drugs worked very well.

After we saw the horrors of drug use, the next topic we discussed was something called VD, or venereal disease. Today, we call this topic sexually transmitted diseases. I had no idea what VD was at the age of 13, but I soon became very aware. We saw movies on the subject of VD. These movies were shown to sailors in the Navy during World War II to warn them of what could happen to them if they had unprotected sex with prostitutes when they got off the ship at their port of call. At that time, I had no idea of what a sexually transmitted disease was, let alone what it looked like when it was on the penis. These films shocked and scared me to the point that I never wanted to have sex if this was what was at risk. At least, that's what I thought at the time.

If the teacher's goal was to scare us into sexual abstinence, then those films were pretty effective, at least in the short run.

After discussing the evils of drugs and sexually transmitted diseases, we then proceeded with the discussion of sex. We were all waiting with much anticipation. Looking back at this educational experience, I find the juxtaposition of the topics interesting. Why would these classes lump our sexual discussion with the subjects of drugs and sexually transmitted diseases? It was communicating a pretty strong negative message about sex on some psychological level to a group of innocent teenage boys. Maybe that's what they intended—an early attempt of teaching abstinence, at least subliminally.

The gym coach's approach to teaching us "men" about sex amounted to a very rudimentary anatomy lesson about male and female reproductive organs and associated drawings. The one element the coach left out in his lecture was how the male's sperm got together with the female egg, the missing link to sexual reproduction. None of the students in my class felt comfortable enough to ask the coach to explain sexual intercourse because he was a very intimidating person, and the whole topic was embarrassing. As a result of this lack of information, we kept asking each other in what female orifice the penis was to go to create a pregnancy. Sexual misinformation and mythology about sexual intercourse went from one classmate to another.

In high school, the only place I heard about sex again was in my biology class. Again, this was a discussion about sexual reproductive anatomy. This discussion was a little more complex than the one lecture I heard from my gym coach back in middle school, but not a whole lot better.

Today, high schools are much more sophisticated in the way they present material about sex. They have had to adjust with the advent of the HIV epidemic and the skyrocketing rate of teen pregnancies.

Some school districts push for an abstinence approach to sex education. An abstinence-only curriculum is a mostly American form of sex education that teaches abstinence from sex and often excludes many other types of sexual and reproductive health education, particularly regarding birth control and safe sex. This type of sex education promotes sexual abstinence until marriage and avoids discussion of the use of contraceptives. Comprehensive sex education, by contrast, covers the use of contraceptives, as well as abstinence. The research evidence does not support the effectiveness of abstinence-only sex education.(2)

After graduating high school, I went to a community college for my first two years of college. The school didn't offer any classes in the area of human sexuality at that time. When I transferred to the University of California–Berkeley in the early 1970s, I thought that maybe a class in human sexuality would be offered, but it didn't exist. After Berkeley, I went to California State University–East Bay for graduate school, and you might think that finally I would get to take a class in human sexuality, but none was available. Soon after that, things did change, and most colleges and universities began offering human sexuality classes. I started teaching my own Human Sexuality class in 1976 at Diablo Valley College in Pleasant Hill, California.

That is how the subject of sex was handled through my past educational experience. I am sure that my experience in some way influenced my own sexuality, as well as the way I teach the subject myself. Your experience may be different, depending on your age and where you went to school, but it's important to understand those past experiences and what roles they played in shaping your own sexual attitudes and beliefs today.

The Peer Group

"Peer pressure is always tough to deal with, especially when it comes to sex. Some teenagers decide to have sexual relationships because their friends think sex is cool. Others feel pressured by the person they are dating. Still others find it easier to give in and have sex than to try to explain why not. Some teenagers get caught up in the romantic feelings and believe having sex is the best way they can prove their love."(3)

Parents find it hard to talk to their kids about sex, religious institutions don't really want to deal with the topic, and the schools have their hands tied by community interests. As a result of the inability of these institutions to effectively tackle the subject of human sexuality, a void of comprehensive sexual information has been created. Where will young, sexually curious adolescents go for sex information? Where teenagers have been going for generations—to their peers. Studies show that details of sexual intercourse, prostitution, and contraception come from a child's peers. The problem with peers being a primary source of sex education is this is where so many of our sexual myths and misconceptions get passed down from one generation to another. Given that young adolescents are hungry for any sexual information that satisfies their thirst for sexual knowledge, they cling to any information they get, whether or not it's correct.

Most teens like to boast that they know what they are talking about when it comes to the subject of sex. They wouldn't want to admit that they might be wrong. Their resource for this knowledge is often an older brother or sister, and of course they assume that the older sibling knows what they are talking about by virtue of their age and all of their personal experience.

"Besides learning from their older siblings, teens learn about sex from all the media sources: music videos, movies, reality shows, beer ads, online porn, prostitutes in video games, sexy doctor shows. Sex is everywhere. And studies show that the more sexual content kids watch and listen to, the earlier they're likely to have sex themselves. In fact, teens report that their main source of information about sex, dating and sexual health comes from what they see and hear in the media. Public health experts say that the media can be an effective sex educator when it includes specific information on birth control methods and sexually transmitted diseases. But in 2005, out of 68% of TV shows that showed steamy sexual content, only 15% discussed risk and responsibility. And it's not just movies and TV: Music, video games, and the Internet are also filled with sexually explicit, often-degrading messages that can shape kids' attitudes about sex."(4)

Males in particular tend to be competitive with each other when it comes to their sexual knowledge. It's this competition that keeps them from admitting they don't know what to do sexually. It basically keeps them sexually ignorant.

In his book, *The New Male Sexuality*, Bernie Zilbergeld quotes an article Bill Cosby wrote for *Playboy* magazine some years ago that best illustrates this concept of male sexual ignorance. In it, Cosby talked about his embarrassment at being a young man, going over to his girlfriend's house to have sex, and not even knowing what sex was. He wrote:

> *"So now, I am walkin' and I'm trying figure out how to do it. And when I get there the most embarrassing thing is gonna be when I have to take my pants down. See, right away then, I am buck naked in front of this girl. Now what happens then? Do you ... do you just ... I don't even know what to do. I'm gonna stand there and she's gonna say, You don't know how to*

> *do it. And I'm gonna say, yes I do, but I forgot. I never thought of her showin me because I'm a man and I don't want her to show me ... I don't want nobody to show me, but I wish somebody would kinda slip me a note."(5)*

The thing is, men are expected to know what to do, even when they are clueless. Some men are so insecure about sex that it takes years before they reach the point where they don't need someone to "slip them a note."(6)

It is with our peer group that early sexual experimentation takes place. It is a normal process of childhood development for sexual exploration to occur between children of the same ages. I am not talking about incest or any form of sexual abuse. That type of behavior is unacceptable. When I was "playing doctor" with my neighborhood friends, everything I did was out of sexual curiosity. "I will show you mine if you show me yours" really had nothing to do with sex because at that age, I didn't really know what the word sex meant. All I knew was that girls had something different "down there," and I was curious to see what that looked like.

When my mother found out what my neighborhood friends and I were up to in our clubhouse in the garage, she was upset and outraged. She yelled at me for doing something "wrong" and punished me as a consequence for my actions. I had such shame and embarrassment for my sexual curiosity, and I am sure that those emotions had a lasting impression on my sexual development.

Dr. Robert Saltzman states on his website that sexual experimentation is a normal part of child development, and that the things children do to investigate their bodies and try to satisfy their developing curiosity about sex are not equivalent in meaning to what those same things would mean if an adult did them.(7)

The Media

Of all the sources of sexual socialization and education, the media is the most influential. Through all the media delivery channels—whether it be the Internet, television, radio, music, movies, or magazines—we as a culture are bombarded with sexual messages that are overt, covert, and subliminal. Subliminal means that we are receiving a message, but it is sent in such a way that we aren't really conscious that our brains are receiving the message. This makes it rather difficult to reject the message outright.

Unless a child lives in a cave, it would be hard for them to escape the media in American culture. I have known parents who want to protect their innocent children from the messages of the media, but usually to no avail because these messages and the media are so pervasive. The communication forms are so powerful—more than we realize—that they can speed up changes that may have taken a lot longer in the past. As a result, there is often a loss of innocence sexually in childhood development.

The media surrounds us—as big business, art, entertainment, and propaganda. To understand the issues and concepts of our time, we must understand both its influence and inspiration. As a culture, we need to develop something called media literacy. Just as we learned in our English literature classes to dissect and analyze printed stories, we need to do the same with the digital media of our time.

American culture today is drenched in sexual messages. As the saying goes, sex is used to sell everything. Given that we are now exposed to an estimated 2500-plus ads per day, the power of these sexual messages and their influence on our youth must not be overlooked. Advertisers use images to get our attention for barely seconds, but that is enough time for our brains to register the image and interpret and register a message. These images appeal to powerful human drives and fantasies and are often used to capture the attention for the purpose of making money. "These images surround us in grocery stores, convenience stores, billboards, magazines, music video, film, and television, to name only a few places."(8)

When we see sexual images in the media, we see perfection. We see images that have been manipulated through computer technology that can create a perfect image of the human body. People don't want to look at images of imperfection because then we have to look at our own imperfections, and that makes us uncomfortable.

The problem with looking at images of humans who always look perfect is that we begin to think we are looking at reality. So reality and fantasy become blurred to the point where we no longer see what is real. People begin to compare their own body image in the mirror to the images embedded in their brains by the media. When this occurs, people are using these unrealistic, fantasy, perfected, computer-generated images as a benchmark for how they should look. Unfortunately, when we use this benchmark for evaluation, it will always lead us to disappointment and frustration. A sense of helplessness and inadequacy ensues because we are being set up for failure.

Are advertisers trying to destroy our self-esteem and self-image? No, they just want us to buy their products, thinking that if we do so, then we can attain these images of perfection. Of course, it's impossible, but we keep trying and keep buying the products. So, advertisers and corporations make money at the expense of our self-esteem and self-image, but it's our fault because we give them the power. So don't be a victim—take your power back, and see through the game of chasing unrealistic physical expectations that the media system and corporations keep putting in your face.

If it is correct that sexual behavior is mostly learned rather than instinctive, then the greatest teacher of sex to modern man has probably been the motion picture. This was true for the 20th century, but today, the Internet and the pornography industry have taken over as the great sex educator for today's youth.

"Although sexual content in the media can affect any age group, adolescents may be particularly vulnerable. Adolescents may be exposed to sexual content in the media during a developmental period when gender roles, sexual attitudes, and sexual behaviors are being shaped. This group may be particularly at risk because the cognitive skills that allow them to critically analyze messages from the media and to make decisions based on possible future outcomes are not fully developed."(9)

What are the psychological effects of learning about sex through today's media, especially via the Internet? It may be too early to truly understand or realize specifically what the long-term impact will be on teens' easy access to pornographic sexual material on the Internet. But one impact that is clear to me is that the experience of emotional intimacy will diminish in future couples' relationships. Examples of healthy intimacy and sensuality are not part of the type of sexuality that exists on the pornographic websites viewed by teens. This is especially true for the male population of young adolescents.

Young males may think the sexual interaction they watch on the pornographic websites is reality. Again, in the media, we have the blurring of boundaries between reality and fantasy. Pornographic sex on the Internet will be mistaken for real life. As inexperienced adolescents, they won't be able to differentiate between the two psychologically. Without a doubt, pornographic sex is acting—it isn't real.

When these teen boys who have been watching sexual interactions on the Internet are in their thirties and married, they will be very disappointed when their wife doesn't want to be some kind of porn star in their bedroom, especially when there is no emotional intimacy or sensuality in the way they make love. I can see a major need for marriage and sex therapists in the future.

Conclusion

Now that we have explored at a basic level the social influences that have shaped our sexual attitudes and behavior, there is so much more to discover. You could write on book on each of these influences. For my purposes, I wanted you to have a general understanding of these influences so you could do your own further research on these topics if you wish.

Just because as children and adolescents we were exposed to these influences does not mean that we can't change or counter the social programming we received. You don't have to be a victim or helpless. You can create a different attitude or approach to sex, despite your socialization. Socialization is a learning process, and what you have learned can be changed. It's not genetic.

Works Cited

1. The Henry J. Kaiser Family Foundation/ABC Television, *Sex in the 90s: 1998 National Survey of Americans on Sex and Sexual Health*, Sept. 1998.
2. http://en.wikipedia.org/wiki/Sex_education_in_the_United_States
3. http://www.iwannaknow.org/teens/relationships/peerpressure.html
4. www.greatschools.org
5. Zilbergeld, Bernie. The New Male Sexuality. New York: Bantam Books, 1999.
6. Keesling, Barbara. Men in Bed: Everything a Woman Needs to Know About the Good, the Bad, and ... New York: Hudson Street Press/Penguin, 2008.
7. http://askdrrobert.dr-robert.com/sexplay.html
8. http://depts.washington.edu/taware/view.cgi?section=s2
9. http://www.ncbi.nlm.nih.gov/pmc/articles/PMC1070813/#ref1

3

Psychological Sexual Development

In the field of psychological study, three areas of human development are generally explored: gender, personality, and sexuality. Each of these can comprise a whole semester of study in upper-division psychology programs. In this chapter, I will just provide a general overview of how we develop sexually using the different psychological theoretical approaches.

If you decide to major in psychology in college, you will see that there isn't just one theoretical approach to explaining how humans develop. If you have a need for one right approach to explain human actions and attitudes, the study of psychology may not fit your personality.

The Freudian-Psychoanalytic Theoretical Approach

Generally, all psychological explanations start with the writings of Sigmund Freud. His theoretical perspective is called the psychoanalytic point of view. He laid the theoretical groundwork for modern psychology. Freud asserts that there is a strong relationship between a child's sexual development and his or her personality traits later in adult life.

Freud maintains that a newborn child is endowed with a certain amount of sexual energy. The child possesses this instinctual sexual energy, which develops in five stages as the child matures. Each of these stages has an associated pleasure zone of the body. The child's passage through the five stages not only determines their sexual functioning as an adult, but their personality development as well.

The first stage of psychosexual development is called the **oral stage**. This stage starts at birth until the age of two years. The baby's mouth is the focus of sexual pleasure. When a baby puts everything in its mouth, including its mother's breast, it experiences pleasure.

Weaning is the key experience in the infant's oral stage of psychosexual development, his first feeling of loss consequent to losing the physical intimacy of feeding at the mother's breast. Yet, weaning increases the infant's awareness that she does not control the environment, and thus learns about delayed gratification, which leads to the formation of the capacities for **independence** (awareness of the limits of the self) and **trust** (behaviors leading to gratification).

The second stage of psychosexual development is known as the **anal stage**. This covers the age from around eighteen months to about three years of age. The child's erogenous zone or pleasure zone of the body changes from its mouth to the anus. Toilet training is the child's key anal-stage experience, occurring at about the age of two years, and results in conflict between the child's need for immediate gratification and the desire for delayed gratification in eliminating bodily wastes and responding to other parental demands.

The third stage of psychosexual development is the phallic stage, covering the ages between three to about six years. During this time, children become aware of their own genitals, which become their primary pleasure zone. They also focus on the bodies of other children and their parents. They satisfy their curiosity through early sexual exploration with their peers by undressing and examining each other's genitals to learn the physical differences between male and female.

It is also in this stage that Freud postulated what he calls the Oedipus complex. He believed that all boys at about age three or four develop unconscious sexual desires for their mothers. They yearn, literally—though unconsciously—to have sexual intercourse with their mothers. However, every boy soon realizes that he cannot have his mother in this way because someone else already does, namely his father. He worries that his father might discover the secret desire he has for his mother. Freud called this worry castration anxiety because the boy is afraid that his father will cut off his penis as punishment for his sexual desire. To reduce this anxiety and conflict, the child decides to identify with his father and emulate him. He sees that he can't take his father on in competition, so instead of fighting him, he wants to become like his father.

Freud also developed a similar theory for girls called the Electra complex. According to this theory, when a girl is about three years old, she realizes that unlike her father, she and her mother don't have penises. Being upset about this situation, she feels "castrated," and develops something that Freud calls penis envy. To make up for this loss, she rejects her mother and wants to identify with her father to obtain his penis, but she sees that she can't because her mother already has ownership. With this realization, she goes back to identifying with her mother, so that when she grows up, she can be with her own husband and his penis.

The next psychosexual stage is called the latency period. It starts at around six years of age and continues until the child moves into puberty. During this period, it seems as if the child's sexual desires and activity become dormant. During this time, children seek out friends of the same sex and don't seem to have much interest in the opposite sex. The child's focus is on sports and developing other life skills.

This could be seen vividly 40 years ago on the playgrounds of elementary schools, but today, because of the influence of the media, I think it has changed. The playground has become much more sexualized compared to the past.

All of these dormant sexual feelings and activity change when the child hits puberty and the sexual hormones come into play. This is called the genital stage, and occurs around the age of 13. This is a time of adolescent sexual experimentation, the successful resolution of which is settling down in a loving one-to-one relationship with another person, usually in our twenties. Sexual instinct is directed to heterosexual pleasure, rather than the self-pleasure that occurred during the phallic stage.

"For Freud, the proper outlet of the sexual instinct in adults was through heterosexual intercourse. Fixation and conflict may prevent this with the consequence that sexual perversions may develop. For example, fixation at the oral stage may result in a person gaining sexual pleasure primarily from kissing and oral sex, rather than sexual intercourse."(1)

Personality and sexual problems occur within the psychoanalytical model when a child fixates at one of these stages. They are unable to move through the stage psychologically with resolution. Their sexual energy has become permanently invested in a particular stage, and therefore, as an adult individual, they display childlike behaviors that are associated with that period of development.

It is believed from a psychoanalytic point of view that if an infant receives too much or too little oral stimulation, it may develop a fixation or a personality trait that is fixated on oral gratification. As adults, these people may focus on activities that involve the mouth, such as overeating, biting the fingernails, smoking, or drinking. According to this theory, these individuals may develop personality traits such as becoming extremely gullible or naive, always following others and never taking the lead, and becoming extremely dependent upon others.

Another example of being stuck in a particular stage and the consequence is when a child's focus becomes receiving pleasure through controlling and eliminating feces: as an adult, they will have the personality traits of being obsessed with control, perfection, and cleanliness. This is often referred to as anal retentive, while anal expulsive is the opposite. Those who are anal expulsive may be extremely disorganized, live in chaos, and create out-of- control situations in their lives.

From the psychoanalytic point of view, all mental, personality, and emotional problems are viewed as having a sexual basis. The treatment to cure these problems is to discover at what stage of development the patient fixated or got stuck in moving on to the next stage of development. When this discovery occurs, the psychological problem will be resolved.

The Biological View of Sexual Development

In addressing human sexual development, one dominant theory is the biological perspective. The biological point of view places a heavy emphasis on the role that hormones play in how an individual will develop sexually in their adult life. The two dominant hormones that influence sexual development are testosterone and estrogen.

These two hormones may be viewed as one of the major driving forces of sexual behavior. Over the past several years, much research has been done in examining the various roles that hormones play in the sexual behavior of humans. Hormones are produced by the gonads (i.e., testes and ovaries), the adrenal cortex, the pituitary gland, and the hypothalamus. In addition, the hormones androgen, estrogen, and progestin all exist in both males and females. They exist in different concentrations, however, within males and females. Males have a higher concentration of androgens, and females have a higher concentration of estrogens and progestin. Incidentally, androgens are responsible for the sexual differentiation of the male reproductive system before birth and the sexual maturation of boys at puberty. Testosterone, a specific androgen, is associated with the male sexual drive and possibly with aggressive behavior.(2)

"Estrogen and progestin, found in higher concentrations within females, regulate the menstrual cycle and are essential for reproduction. The relationship of these hormones to the female sexual drive and behavior are unclear. Hormone levels are usually correlated with sexual behavior, but in humans this is not necessarily true because of intervening variables. Thus, an individual may be physiologically ready to participate in sexual behavior, but does not because of factors that supersede any biological reason."(3)

There are two periods in a child's life where sex hormones play a significant role in shaping his or her sexual development in adulthood. The first critical period is prenatally, or shortly after birth.

The hormonal theory of sexuality holds that just as exposure to certain hormones plays a role in fetal sex differentiation, such exposure also influences the sexual orientation that emerges later in the adult. Differences in brain structure that come about from hormones and genes interacting on developing brain cells are believed to be the basis of sex differences in countless behaviors, including sexual orientation.(4)

The second critical period when sex hormones play a major role in shaping our sexual development is at the onset of puberty. In girls, it starts between the ages of ten and 14, when the pituitary gland starts producing hormones that stimulate the production of the sex hormones by the ovaries. These sex hormones are estrogen and progesterone. They bring about profound bodily changes—called secondary sex characteristics—that occur during puberty. Breasts begin to develop, hips and thighs widen, and pubic and underarm hair develops. The ovaries start producing eggs, and menstruation starts.

Boys also go through physical changes at the onset of puberty. Usually between the ages of 12 and 15, the pituitary gland releases hormones that stimulate the production of testosterone in the boy's testes. When the testosterone is released, the boy starts to develop secondary characteristics. His voice deepens, and hair begins to grow on his face and body. The genitals develop, along with pubic hair. Sperm is being produced, and he experiences wet dreams.

Sexual problems can occur, despite the presence of an adequate supply of hormones. This illustrates the point that sexual development cannot be looked at apart from social context. Biological factors play a significant role in sexual development. They operate within the context of other psychological and social factors that affect development.

The Cognitive-Experimental Viewpoint

In the 1970s, University of Massachusetts psychologist Seymour Epstein, PhD, developed his "cognitive-experiential self-theory." In it, he points out that human beings process information through two systems: Just as we learn things consciously all the time—the cognitive part of the theory—we also learn things experientially, without realizing we've learned them. "Intuition is just the things we've learned without realizing we've learned them. And sometimes they're useful. Sometimes they're maladaptive," Epstein says.(5)

Looking at sexual development from this point of view, sexual functioning requires that humans have normal contact with other humans. In our developmental process, we are constantly receiving cognitive messages regarding sexual dos and don'ts. This process starts early in childhood, and by the time we are adolescents, we are bombarded with sexual messages. Some of these messages are delivered subliminally, some are overt, and others are covert. This is the cognitive part of development.

When a baby isn't held and touched and is ignored over long periods of time, most likely this child won't develop into a functional sexual adult. The adult will be very uncomfortable with touching and affection with another person. He may develop a type of hypersensitivity to physical touch that makes affection very uncomfortable. Not being able to touch another person highly restricts the enjoyment of the sexual experience.

The playful activity of children roughhousing is a necessary precursor to successful sexual behavior. This is their way of getting comfortable with physical contact with the other members of their species.

"Loving touch also serves many purposes. Through repeated animal and human experiments over a 50-year period, medical researchers, such as Bowlby, Harlow, Hansen, Montagu and many others, have stated that touch is vital for the growth of several 'physiological systems' and is vital for the foundation for healthy, loving, relationships."(6) "Moreover, Montagu points out from his research that loving touch is an essential behavioral need just as breathing is a physical need. From this, a newborn is made to 'grow and develop' receiving nurturing, maternal touch and sustaining that form of touch with others throughout its life."(7) "Furthermore, the development of self-esteem is at least partly based on the amount of loving touch one receives."(8)

"Not only is being touched during infancy critical to sexual development, it's also critical during adolescence. In the beginning of the teenage years, parents cease to touch their children. This is partly due to their discomfort with the physical developmental changes within their children. This might account for the hyper sexual activity of teenagers who focus on their peers to satisfy their need for touch and sex as a vehicle to get held."(9)

We take all of our sexual cognitive development and our beliefs out into the world and experiment with what we have learned. This experimentation also shapes our sexual development relevant to the culture to which we are exposed.

The cognitions or attitudes an individual possesses provide a mental structure or a set of constraints on their capacity for sexual expression. A young boy learns pretty quickly that if he touches a girl's breast just because he feels like it, it won't be something that he does again. He experiments with his behavior and then learns the cognitive belief that his behavior is not acceptable.

When young children "play doctor" with each other, this is another experiment to learn about differences between the sexes. This is a component in their sexual development. From this experimental experience, they will develop cognitive beliefs regarding sexual behavior. When my mother caught me playing doctor with the girl next door, I learned that this was not something I wanted to do again. A cognitive constraint was put into place as far as my sexual development was concerned.

Social Learning Theory of Sexual Development

According to social learning theory, we learn by observing the behaviors of others and by interacting with them. Children have models in their lives such as parents or peers who can either inhibit certain sexual behaviors or have a disinhibitory effect. Children look at the behaviors of parents, not so much to learn how to make sexual responses as to determine when such responses are appropriate.

As the founder of social learning theory, Albert Bandura stated in 1977: "Learning would be exceedingly laborious, not to mention hazardous, if people had to rely solely on the effects of their own actions to inform them what to do. Fortunately, most human behavior is learned observationally through modeling: from observing others one forms an idea of how new behaviors are performed, and on later occasions this coded information serves as a guide for action."(10) It becomes critical from the social learning theory that we interact with our own species in order to develop sexually.

Social learning theory believes that we can learn by seeing the rewards and punishments that others receive for their actions, without having to experience them personally. Individuals learn about their own sexuality by first imitating the behavior of others and then acting, after having developed an anticipation of the potential results. In the field of sexuality, this theory has been applied to sexual violence. It is not uncommon for erotic films or magazines to show a woman enjoying the advances of a sexually aggressive man, even if she may at first deny him. It has become a concern that exposure of adolescent boys to such scenarios may send the message that women are sexually aroused by aggressive, perhaps even violent or assaultive, methods.(11)

Besides the extreme aggressive modeling as it relates to sex that young male adolescents witness through the images of the media, they are also exposed to very explicit sexual behavior in general, primarily through the Internet and all the pornography they can access. Gail Dines states in her book, *Pornland*, that "the average age of first viewing porn is now 11.5 years for boys, and with the advent of the Internet, it's no surprise that young people are consuming more porn than ever. But, as Dines shows, today's porn is strikingly different from yesterday's Playboy. As porn culture has become absorbed into pop culture, a new wave of entrepreneurs are creating porn that is even more hard-core, violent, sexist, and racist. To differentiate their products in a glutted market, producers have created profitable niche products—like teen sex, torture porn, and gonzo—in order to entice a generation of desensitized users."(12)

This influence on male sexual development may also have a tremendous effect on women's sexuality. "This hypersexualization has put pressure on women to look and act like they just tumbled out of the pages of *Maxim* or *Cosmopolitan*. Whether it be thongs peeping out of low-slung jeans, revealing their 'tramp stamp,' their waxed pubic area, or their desire to give the best blow job ever to the latest hookup, young women and girls, it seems, are increasingly celebrating their 'empowering' sexual freedom by trying to look and act the part of a porn star," writes Dines.(13)

The long-term effects of this type of sexual development through exposure to the Internet are yet to be determined, but I think it will create problems within the context of a serious long-term relationship.

We learn through our sexual experiments as we develop as children. From our early sexual experiments, we realize what acceptable behavior within our culture is. We develop a set of cognitions that provides us with a limiting set of constraints on our capacity for sexual expression. A boy learns fairly quickly that touching a girl's breast will elicit a negative reaction.

Works Cited

1. http://www.simplypsychology.org/saul-mcleod.html
2. Molina, Ludwin. *Human Sexuality*. California State University, Northridge, spring 1999.
3. http://en.wikipedia.org/wiki/Prenatal_hormones_and_sexual_orientation#cite_note-Garcia-Falgueras-Swaab-SexualHormonesBrain-p24-1
4. "What we know without knowing how, Psychologists are working to understand our split-second, unconscious judgments and deductions." Lea Winerman. *American Psychologist Monitor* staff, March 2005, Vol. 36, No. 3.
5. http://www.touchangels.com/articles/critical.html
6. Montagu, A. *The Human Significance of the Skin*, 3rd ed. New York: Harper & Row Publishers, 1986.
7. Andersen, J. E., Andersen, P. A., & Lusting, L. W. (1987). "Opposite Sex Touch Avoidance: A National Replication and Extension." *Journal of Nonverbal Behavior*, Vol. 2, pp. 89–109.
8. www.touchangels.com/articles/critical.html
9. http://psychology.about.com/od/developmentalpsychology/a/sociallearning.htm
10. http://online.missouri.edu/exec/data/courses/2393/public/lessono1.asp
11. Dines, Gail. *Pornland: How Porn Has Hijacked Our Sexuality*. Boston: Beacon Press, 2010.
12. Dines, Gail. *Pornland: How Porn Has Hijacked Our Sexuality*. Boston: Beacon Press, 2010.

4

Sexual Anatomy

When I first started teaching sexual anatomy, I wondered how I could make this topic interesting for my students. Anatomy sounds so dry—just describing the sexual anatomical parts of the human body. Over the years, I have discovered that there is a whole psychological element to human sexual anatomy that can have a major impact on a couple's sexual experience.

Do you fully understand your own body from a sexual point of view, how it functions, and why you have certain sexual responses? Do you know the locations of your sexual anatomy? These might sound like strange questions to ask, but from my experience, few men and women fully understand their bodily functions, particularly the anatomy and physiology of their sexual organs.

Why is there such ignorance regarding sexual anatomy? When the subject of sexual anatomy is brought out in the open, most of us feel embarrassed. When the terms penis or vagina are used in common discussion, people feel uncomfortable. We don't have this kind of emotional reaction to any other part of the human anatomy, but when sexual organs are mentioned, people feel embarrassed.

We are taught from a very early age that we are not supposed to talk about our sexual anatomy. We are told that these are our "private parts," and we are supposed to keep them hidden. An innocent child starts to interpret from his parents that there is something wrong with his sexual anatomy. He starts to develop a certain amount of shame; hence, the emotion of embarrassment when these terms are discussed. Parents don't even use the correct anatomical names; they make up euphemisms like pee-pee or other names.

All of this uneasiness surrounding the discussion of sexual anatomical parts leaves many children and adults ignorant about their own sexual anatomy. People just don't talk about this subject, and as a result fall prey to a great deal of misinformation or sexual myths. Because we don't know what is true as a child, we tend to believe what someone's older brother or sister says, because we want to know something. Of course, we don't check out the reliability of the source. When we are kids, an older teen represents an authority, whatever the topic. In reality, they are probably just passing down the same myths they heard, and the cycle just continues from one generation to the next.

I remember when I was being trained as a sex therapist at the age of 24. I had to learn to work through my own uneasiness using the correct sexual anatomical names like vagina and penis without turning red with embarrassment. It was called desensitization. It would be pretty difficult to help patients with their sex lives or stand up in front of students if I weren't comfortable with the subject matter myself.

One of my goals in this chapter is to address the many sexual anatomical myths that are out there and relay the correct information. You may ask how this will make you a better lover. It's hard to be an effective lover if you don't know about your own specific anatomical sexual parts and how they function, as well as your partner's.

When an individual is inhibited about their sexuality, much of this inhibition is created by fear and anxiety. Often, what causes this fear is an individual's lack of knowledge. Hopefully, studying sexual anatomy will give you accurate knowledge of yourself and your partner and will result in less inhibition about exploring your own sexuality in general.

In my discussion of sexual anatomy, I also want to emphasize how one's anatomy impacts an individual's experience of sexual pleasure. I will point out the concentration of nerve endings in each body part, because understanding nerve cell concentration has an impact on the degree of pleasure the mind experiences.

By the time a person reaches their early twenties, most of what they have learned about sexual anatomy relates to one topic: sexual reproduction. This is what we are taught in our education system from elementary school through high school, and even in college. What is not taught is how to experience sexual pleasure and what can get in its way. I won't be discussing sexual anatomy as it relates to sexual reproduction in any detail, as I think that topic has been covered in biology and health classes in our public school systems.

The general meaning of intercourse is communication. The question is, how can communication occur without basic knowledge about our sexual anatomy?

Female External Sexual Anatomy

When discussing sexual anatomy, I will first discuss the external anatomy and then the internal parts for both sexes. The term used to describe the overall area of external female genitalia is the word vulva, which takes its meaning from the Latin word for covering. Many anatomical names come from Latin, and the psychological meanings can be interpreted from these words.

The vulva is a collective term encompassing the external anatomical parts: the mons veneris, the labia minor, the labia major, the clitoris, and the vaginal and urethral openings. Another Latin name for the vulva is the pudendum, which means "something to be ashamed of." This reflects many women's attitudes about their genitalia. When the women's liberation movement started back in the 1970s, it wanted to change this attitude that women had about their own bodies and instead embrace the positive aspects of their own sexual anatomy.

When discussing sexual anatomy, I can use the clinical terms or the slang terms used in common vernacular. A variety of slang expressions are used for the vulva: terms like box, beaver, bush, pussy, snatch, fur burger, twat, quim, wahoo, muff, and honeypot. What kinds of messages do these terms communicate? How do you feel when you hear or see them in print? Most seem derogatory and demeaning to women, reflecting men's historical attitudes toward women on a sexual level.

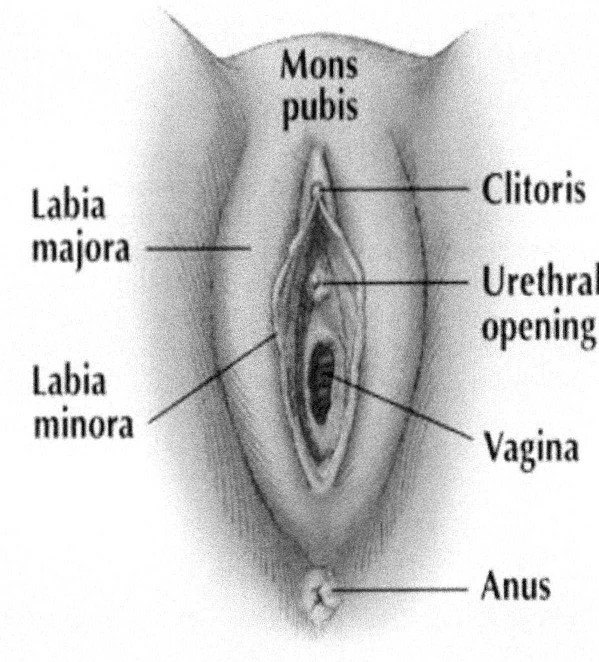

Figure 1: Female external sex organs. Copyright © Schirly (CC BY-SA 3.0) at http://commons.wikimedia.org/wiki/File:Vagina_1.jpg

Mons Veneris

The mons veneris takes its name from the Latin, meaning "the mound of Venus," the Roman goddess of love. The mons veneris is a soft, fatty pad that is covered with pubic hair. The size of the mons veneris varies with the general level of hormones and body fat. After puberty, it is covered with pubic hair and enlarges in size from its pre puberty state. It protects the pubic bone during intercourse. This area has numerous nerve endings, and many women find that gentle stimulation of this area is highly pleasurable.

When a girl reaches puberty, her body produces rising levels of the sex hormones known as androgens, and as a result, secondary sex characteristics begin to develop, one of which is pubic hair. During this time, the skin of the mons veneris begins to produce thicker and rougher, often curlier, hair with a faster growth rate. The color and texture of the pubic hair is related to genetic factors.

What is the purpose of pubic hair? One belief is that the hair that grows around the genitals and under the arms lock in sexually stimulating scents called pheromones. Some people can detect these scents and find that it can increase their desire. Others don't notice anything or find the odor offensive. Some people believe that pubic hair keeps our genitals warm. Others believe that the purpose of pubic hair is to prevent dirt from entering the vagina. This is not so much of an issue in modern times.

Today, there are divergent attitudes about the presence of female pubic hair. For many, less is better, compared to the early 1970s, when hair was everywhere. I believe that how much pubic hair women have today is driven by the pornography industry and what young men watch, and these standards filter down into real life.

The Labia Majora

Some slang terms for this area include the bearded clam, snappers, jaws, or nut breakers. These labels show a certain paranoia from a male viewpoint that somehow a woman's genitals can hurt them or even trap them, which is related to a myth that I will discuss later in the physiology chapter.

The labia majora are more correctly called the large or outer lips. The labia majora start at the thigh and extend inward, surrounding the rest of the vulva. The outer edges are hair covered, and the inner edges are smooth. The skin of the outer lips is rich in blood vessels, and darker than the skin of the thighs. During arousal the labia majora swell and become even darker. They are supplied with nerve endings that contribute to sexual arousal. Prior to adolescence, the outer lips come together, covering the rest of the vulva; after puberty, the lips are slightly parted, showing some of the labia minora.

The Labia Minora

The labia minora are the "small" lips of the female reproductive system and are, at most, two inches wide. They vary greatly in size, shape, and form. The labia minora are found on the inner side of the labia majora and surround both the openings of the urethra and the vagina. The meeting point of both the labia minora is the clitoris, which forms the hood. The labia minora do not have any pubic hair, but they are well endowed with blood vessels. During sexual arousal, the labia minora swell due to the increase in blood flow, and they change in color.

The labia minora give off natural glandular secretions that lubricate the area during sexual arousal. This lubrication is not to be confused with vaginal lubrication. There are also sweat glands located in the skin of the labia minora that provide a natural aroma.

Bartholin's Glands

The Bartholin's glands are located at the base of the minor lips. With prolonged stimulation, these glands provide the inner surface of the labia with a few drops of mucus-like fluid to provide vaginal lubrication. Bartholin's glands secrete relatively minute amounts (one or two drops) of fluid when a woman is sexually aroused. These droplets of fluid were once believed to be important for lubricating the vagina, but research from Masters and Johnson demonstrates that vaginal lubrication comes from deeper within the vagina. The fluid may slightly moisten the labial opening of the vagina, serving to make contact with this sensitive area more comfortable for the woman during intercourse. It's not uncommon for these glands to become infected and lead to an abscess that must be removed.

The Clitoris

When I was in high school in the late 1960s, I never knew what the clitoris was—the word was never mentioned. By the early 1970s, it became the most discussed anatomical part of a woman's body. The clitoris was seen as a way for a woman to take ownership of her own sexuality. The clitoris was, after all, a major source of feminist consciousness-raising in the 1970s. This tiny organ took on a significant role in the sexual politics of the time. The clitoris was seen as a direct path for a woman to experience her full orgasmic potential through direct or indirect clitoral stimulation.

Throughout history, the clitoris—and its great potential—has been lost and found over and over again. In spotlighting the clitoris, women's liberation proponents exposed oppressive social untruths about female biology. They countered the old Freudian myth of the vagina as the exclusive natural source of a true "mature" woman's pleasure and the clitoris as a "girlish phase."(1)

Slang terms referring to the clitoris include clit, little man in a boat, love button, and love bud. The clitoris has the fewest number of slang terms when compared to other parts of the female sexual anatomy. This may have to do with the fact that many people may not even know of its existence, although this has changed a great deal in the past 40 years.

The clitoris is similar to a male penis anatomically, except it does not have a urethra running through its center. The body of the clitoris consists of tiny spongy tissue, which fills with blood during sexual arousal, resulting in a doubling or tripling in size. The clitoris has a head, or glans, which forms the tip of the clitoris, the most sensitive area. The clitoris is completely covered by a hood, except for the head.

The clitoris is simply a bundle of nerves—8,000 nerve fibers, to be precise. That's the highest concentration of nerve fibers found anywhere on the body, including the fingertips, lips, and tongue, and twice the number of nerves located in the penis. It doesn't get any more sensitive than that. The glans of the clitoris is so sensitive that touching it directly is almost painful, and therefore women may prefer circuitous stimulation of the shaft or the entire mons area.

The sole purpose of the clitoris is to transmit sensations to the female brain. Its function is all about sexual pleasure. It is not a necessary part of sexual reproduction. This wasn't taught in the past, perhaps as a way to keep women from knowing about their own sexuality, except as it related to producing children.

In parts of northeast Africa, the Near East, Southeast Asia, and among some aboriginal groups in South America and Australia, clitoridectomy is practiced, also known as female genital mutilation. The clitoris and labia are removed, often under the most unsanitary conditions and in a crude fashion, and generally against the will of the young girls who are the victims of this procedure. Clitoridectomy is a deplorable practice. It is, among other things, an extremely painful, traumatizing mutilation of young girls that leaves them permanently disfigured and deprives them of sexual enjoyment.

What is the rationale for this torture? The practice is often cited as a puberty rite in late childhood or early adolescence. In some cultures, the removal of the clitoris is believed to keep a girl chaste because the clitoris is sensitive to sexual stimulation. It is feared that girls will otherwise be consumed with sexual desire. Some groups in rural Egypt and in the northern Sudan, however, perform clitoridectomies primarily as a social custom that has been passed down through the generations from ancient times or because they perceive it as part of their faith in Islam, although the Koran itself does not require it.(2)

The Hymen

The hymen is the thin piece of tissue that partially blocks the entrance to the vagina. It is sometimes called the maidenhead or cherry. Named after the Greek god of marriage, it has no known biological function. Although some girls are born without a hymen, most have one, and the hymen varies in size and shape from woman to woman.

A common misconception about the hymen is that it is inside the vagina. It is actually a mucous membrane that is part of the vulva, the external genital organs. The hymen is formed from a layer of tissue that develops in the early stages of fetal development when there is no opening in the vagina at all. This thin layer of tissue conceals the vagina, but usually divides incompletely prior to birth, forming the hymen. Over the centuries, the hymen has been one of the most discussed parts of female sexual anatomy. Its presence was seen as an indicator as to whether or not a young woman was a virgin. But it is a scientific fact that the hymen can be separated for reasons quite unconnected to sexual intercourse. It can separate when the body is stretched strenuously, as in athletics; by inserting a tampon during menstruation; through masturbation; and sometimes it separates for no apparent reason.

A separated hymen is not an indication of having had intercourse, nor can it prove a loss of virginity. "In fact, some women must have their hymen surgically removed before the birth of their first child because it is so flexible or small that it remains intact during intercourse."(3)

Generally, the hymen is perforated to allow for monthly menstrual flow. The hymen does not provide protection from getting pregnant. If any sperm gets near the hymen, they may be able to pass through the membrane because of the microscopic openings that make up the surface of the hymen. This is also true of sexually transmitted diseases.

The Breasts

In our culture, female breasts are seen as highly sexualized external parts of the female anatomy, but on a biological level, they are not sexual at all. They aren't even a part of the sexual reproduction system. They are technically called secondary sex characteristics, which occur as a girl moves into the puberty stage of development. Her breasts develop as a result of increasing levels of the hormone estrogen in her bloodstream.

Breasts also go by many slang terms such as milk jugs, tatas, melons, and boobs. They are mammary glands that, in the female mammal, produce milk for the sustenance of her young. Each breast consists of 15 to 20 milk-producing glands connected to ducts, which lead to the nipple.

It is common for one breast to be slightly larger than the other. What gives breasts their consistency and creates their size is fatty tissue that is loosely packed between the milk-producing

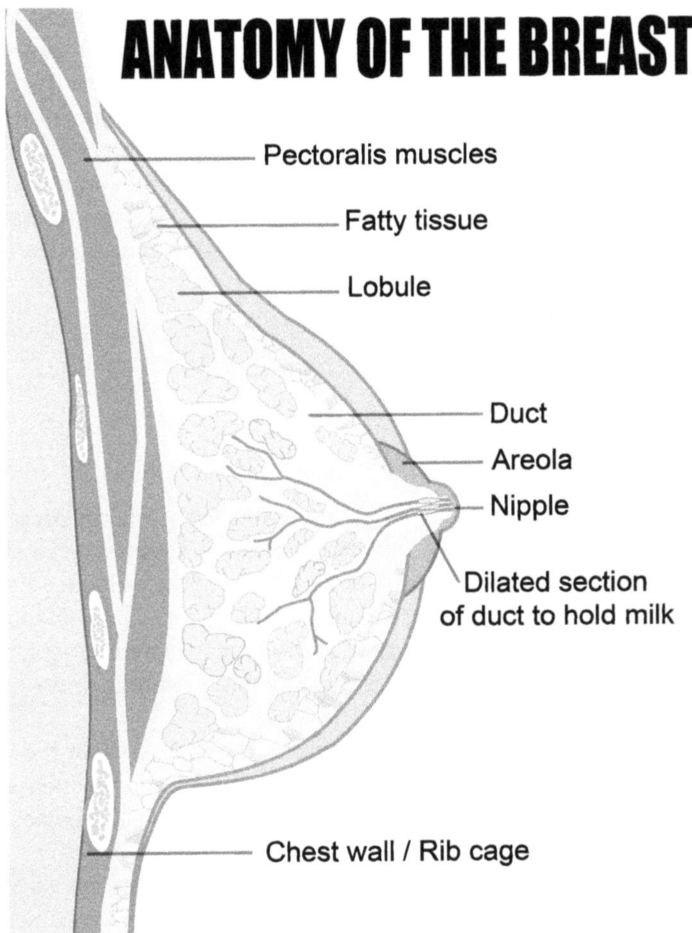

Figure 2: Breast anatomy. Copyright © 2012 Depositphotos/roxanabalint.

glands. Our culture is preoccupied with the size of the female breast.

The general belief in our culture is that the bigger the breasts are, the better. For many girls and women, their sense of their sexuality and physical self-esteem is psychologically attached to the size of their breasts. From an anatomical point of view, there is no correlation between the size and shape of a woman's breasts and her sensitivity to pleasure. Large, natural breasts or those enhanced through plastic surgery don't have a greater number of nerve endings to transport sensations to the brain. Larger breasts just have more fat cells or silicone in them, without any increase in nerve endings. They don't receive more pleasurable sensations.

What makes breasts sexual in our culture is the psychological meaning that we place on them. Many of us are conditioned in our adolescence to believe that the female breast is something sexual. In our culture, men are encouraged by their peers and the media to look at breasts and to feel them. Breasts become objects of men's own sexual pleasure. We check them out in magazines and at the beach, or on the Internet. Discussing women's breasts and looking at them is a way for males to bond with each other. On the other side, adolescent girls with large breasts may be uncomfortable with all this attention. Teenage girls with smaller breasts may feel inadequate and unattractive, affecting their sexual self-esteem. In other cultures and countries, the female breast is just a part of a woman's body and has no particular relationship to sex. I remember going to the beach at a Club Med, which is a French company, in the Bahamas and Mexico, and women of all ages were topless. It was no big deal. It doesn't have the same sexual charge that it does in America, perhaps because other cultures don't have the same conditioning that we have in America regarding breasts.

Internal Female Sexual Anatomy

The Vagina

The vagina, which in Latin means literally sheath or scabbard, is a fibromuscular tubular tract leading from the uterus to the exterior of the female body. In a non-aroused state, the vagina is three to five inches in length. During sexual arousal, the vagina expands in both length and width. Its elasticity allows it to stretch during sexual intercourse and during childbirth. The vagina connects the vulva to the cervix of the deep uterus. If the woman stands upright, the vaginal tube points in an upward-backward direction and forms an angle of slightly more than 45 degrees with the uterus and the small of the back.

The vagina has several functions in a mature female. The first function the vagina provides is a duct for menstrual flow when a woman menstruates. The second function is to receive the penis during intercourse to help with sexual reproduction. And third, it provides a canal for the birth of a child.

Keep in mind that the vagina is a "potential" space, meaning that the walls of the vagina are normally in contact with each other. In other words, they are touching unless something is inserted between them; contrary to what most anatomy illustrations depict—and what a lot of men think—the vagina isn't a hole or cavity inside the body. When something enters the vagina, the body must make room for it, no matter how small or large it may be. Knowing the concept of potential space is important if you want to be a sensitive lover, especially if you are a man. Just because you are ready for sex and have an erection, it doesn't automatically mean that your lover is ready for penetration.

The walls of the vagina are actually made up of three types of tissue. The inside wall is called the mucosa and is similar to the inside of your mouth. Just below the mucosa is a layer of tissue that can fill with blood. This is the erectile tissue, which swells when a woman is sexually aroused. The deepest layer is a coat of muscle. This muscular coat is a wrap of tissue that can relax or constrict.(4)

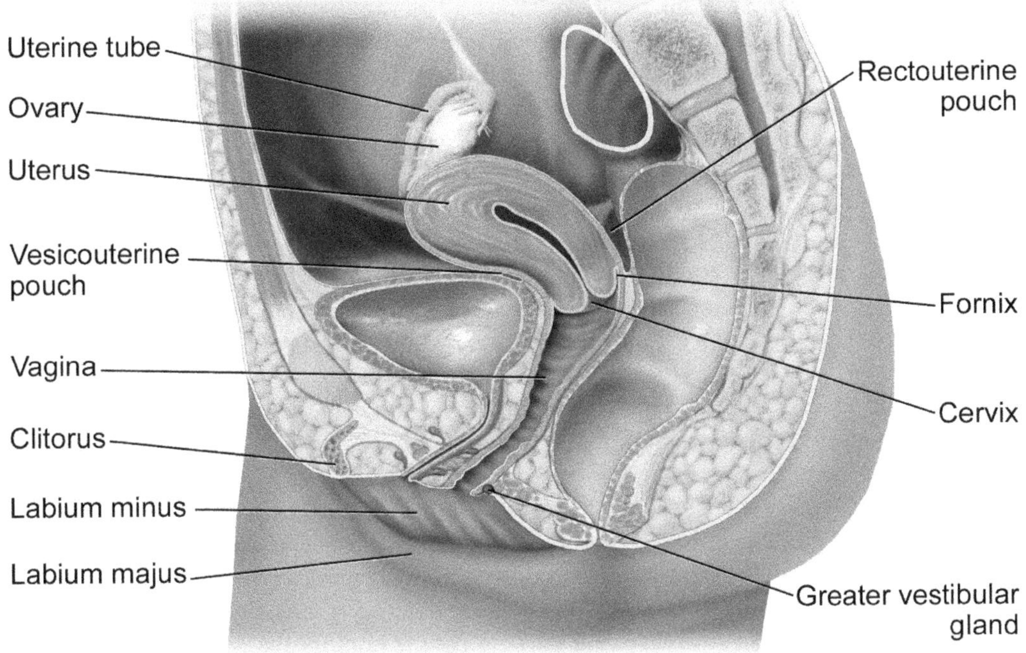

Figure 3: Female reproductive system. Copyright © BruceClaus (CC by 3.0) at http://commons.wikimedia.org/wiki/File:Blausen_0400_FemaleReproSystem_02.png.

Vaginal lubrication is a fluid that is naturally produced in a woman's vagina. For a long time until Masters and Johnson did their research, the source of vaginal lubrication was unclear. Their findings described the mechanisms of vaginal lubrication, debunking the earlier widely held notion that vaginal lubrication originated from the cervix. Vaginal lubrication or moistness is present at all times, but production increases significantly during a woman's sexual arousal in anticipation of sexual intercourse. Without vaginal lubrication, sexual intercourse would be painful to the woman, and sometimes, artificial lubricants must be used to augment insufficient natural lubrication. While plasma seepage from vaginal walls due to vascular engorgement is considered to be the chief lubrication source, the Bartholin's glands—located slightly below and to the left and right of the introitus (opening of the vagina)—also secrete mucus to augment vaginal wall secretions.

Americans have been misled about sexual lubrication, writes medical author Michael Castleman.(5) In the 1960s, pioneering sex researchers William Masters, MD, and Virginia Johnson describe vaginal lubrication as one aspect of initial sexual arousal in women. They maintain that the vagina produces lubrication fairly quickly as a woman becomes aroused. But for many perfectly normal women, vaginal lubrication takes much longer to appear, and when it does, there may not be much of it.

To make matters worse, the erotic stories in such sex publications as *Penthouse* magazine imply that every woman self-lubricates like Niagara Falls at the wink of an alluring eye: "Just being near Bill made my panties wet. ..." Not only is this way off the mark, but it has also led to a destructive corollary, the notion that if a woman does not produce much natural lubrication, she is neither turned on by her lover nor committed to the relationship.

Instant gushing lubrication may happen to some women. But it's much more common for a woman to feel committed to her relationship and erotically aroused by her lover and still not self-lubricate much, if at all.

The mechanics of vaginal lubrication occur when a woman is sexually aroused and there is a subsequent increase of blood flow to the vaginal walls and they become engorged with blood. This engorgement, or vasocongestion, creates pressure that causes the mucus lining to secrete fluid. How much fluid is secreted depends on several factors, including the woman's age.

Before a girl reaches puberty, the walls of her vagina are very thin. Once she enters puberty and large amounts of estrogen are introduced into her body, the walls of her vagina thicken with an increase of the blood vessels. The increase in the vascular makeup of her vaginal walls allows her to lubricate. This all changes when a woman reaches menopause. The walls of her vagina become thin again, and the amount of natural lubrication is greatly reduced.

The vagina is surrounded by the pubococcygeus muscle, more commonly known as the PC muscle. The PC muscle is richly supplied with nerves, and during involuntary or voluntary contracting during intercourse, which increases the sensation of pleasure for the woman and her partner. The PC muscle expands during a woman's pregnancy to accommodate the size of the fetus. Kegel exercises are recommended for pregnant women to help strengthen their PC muscle to help make the delivery easier. Kegels are also recommended to rebuild the strength of the PC muscle after delivery.

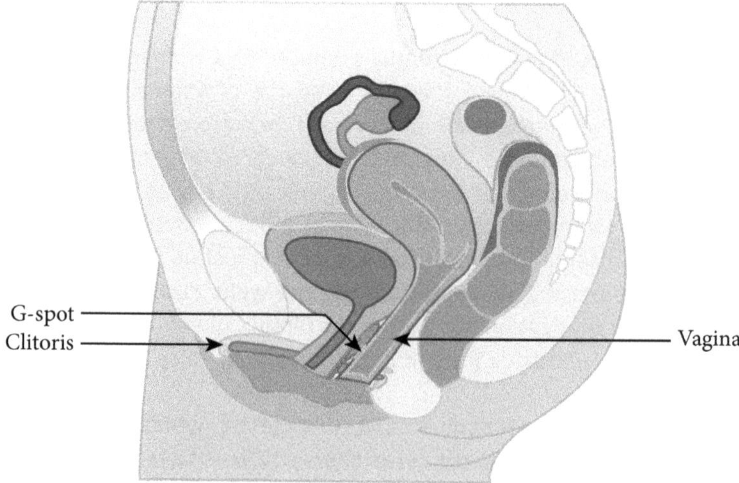

Figure 4: G-spot anatomy. Copyright © Tsaitgaist (CC BY-SA 3.0) at Adapted from: http://commons.wikimedia.org/wiki/File:Female_anatomy_with_g-spot-en.svg

One of the more controversial areas of female internal sexual anatomy has been the subject of the Gräfenberg spot, often called the G-spot, within the vagina. The G-spot is a bean-shaped area typically located one to three inches up the front (anterior) vaginal wall, between the vaginal opening and the urethra. Many women report that it is an erogenous zone, which, when stimulated, can lead to strong sexual arousal and powerful orgasms. The G-spot is a sensitive area that may be part of the "female prostate."

The term G-spot was coined by Frank Addiego and others in 1981, after the German gynecologist Ernst Gräfenberg, even though Gräfenberg's 1940s research was dedicated to urethral stimulation and not internal vaginal wall stimulation. The concept entered popular culture after the publication of *The G Spot and Other Recent Discoveries About Human Sexuality* by Ladas et al. in 1982, but was criticized immediately by leading gynecologists.(6) They denied its existence, as it is not easily found when a woman is not aroused, and autopsy studies missed this. After the G-spot was demonstrated for their observation, they changed their minds. While not disputing vaginal responsiveness to stimulation, some gynecologists and doctors continue to be skeptical of the existence of a distinct anatomical feature in the G-spot rub zone.

Myths About the Vagina

One common myth associated with the vagina is a belief that the deeper that stimulation occurs within the vagina during sexual intercourse, the more pleasure a woman will experience. I have seen this myth expressed in a bumper sticker that reads "Divers do it deeper." Pornography is loaded with examples about "doing it deeper" and how women want this kind of stimulation during intercourse. The belief that deeper is better may be true on a male psychological or fantasy level, but based on the female anatomy, nothing could be further from the truth.

The anatomical fact is that the inner two-thirds of the vagina have very few nerve endings compared to the outer third. With deeper stimulation, the pleasure a woman experiences is reduced, unless she is able to receive greater clitoral contact. If the inner two-thirds of the vagina were well endowed with nerve endings, imagine how much more painful the experience of childbirth would be for a woman.

It's a male fantasy to think that the vagina is the anatomical center of a woman's experience of sexual pleasure. It's not that vaginal stimulation isn't pleasurable; it is, but the majority of nerve endings are located in the clitoris, not the vagina.

Another myth about the vagina is that it needs to be kept clean with soap and water or the use of specially designed douches. The vagina is actually a self-cleansing organ with naturally occurring bacteria that destroy harmful odor-causing bacteria. Vaginal problems occur when the healthy bacteria are destroyed by using body washes, soaps, or douches.

Is douching healthy? Simply stated, the answer is no. Regular vaginal douching changes the delicate chemical balance of the vagina and can make a woman more susceptible to infection. Douching can introduce new bacteria into the vagina, which can spread up through the cervix, uterus, and fallopian tubes. Researchers have found that women who douche regularly experience more vaginal irritation and infections such as bacterial vaginosis, along with an increased number of sexually transmitted diseases.(7)

Another popular story associated with the vagina is about its size relative to the penis. Some believe that women who are small in stature must have smaller vaginas compared to larger women. A woman may believe she has a smaller vagina due to her skeletal frame and so may think that her partner's penis will cause her pain during intercourse.

The truth is that all vaginas are one general size—regardless of a woman's skeletal frame. A woman may be concerned that her vagina is too large for her partner's penis. She worries that this will lead to a decrease in sensitivity and stimulation to adequately satisfy her partner sexually. This issue is not related to vaginal size, but to the condition of her PC muscle. If she exercises and conditions her PC muscle through the use of Kegel exercises, this condition should be corrected.

One last myth associated with the vagina is the idea that it is able to trap a penis during intercourse. This happens between dogs when they have intercourse, but not humans. It's one of those urban legends floating out there among the uneducated. There might be some sensation of this when a male is fully erect and his partner's PC muscle is tight, but once the male starts to lose his erection, his penis is going to slide out of her vagina, no matter how hard her PC muscle is contracting.

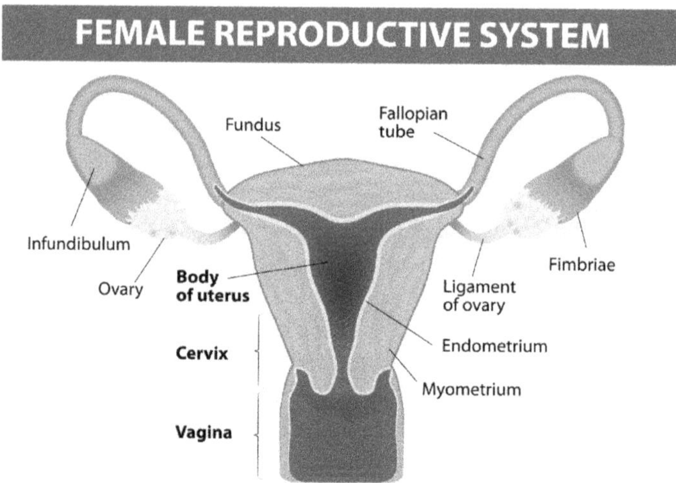

Figure 5: G-spot anatomy. Copyright © Tsaitgaist (CC BY-SA 3.0) at Adapted from: http://commons.wikimedia.org/wiki/File:Female_anatomy_with_g-spot-en.svg

The Uterus

The cervix is the lower third of the uterus, forming the neck of the uterus and opening into the vagina. The narrow opening of the cervix is called the os. The cervical os allows menstrual blood to flow out from the vagina during menstruation. During pregnancy the cervical os closes to help keep the fetus in the uterus until birth. Another important function of the cervix occurs during labor when the cervix dilates, or widens, to allow the passage of the fetus from the uterus to the vagina.

For women, having regular Pap smears is imperative to detect early changes to the cervical cells, which may lead to cervical cancer; however, the majority of abnormal Pap smear results are due to inflammation or infection.(8)

The uterus looks like an inverted pear when it doesn't have a fetus developing inside. In a pre-pregnancy state, it measures three inches long and three inches wide at the top. Three inches is rather small when you compare that to how much the uterus expands when a fetus is growing within the uterus. No other organ expands as much as the uterus during pregnancy. Generally, the uterus is perpendicular to the vagina, but sometimes it is tilted, causing pain for a woman when she has intercourse in certain positions.

The lining of the uterine cavity is called the endometrium. Shedding of the functional endometrial lining is responsible for menstrual bleeding (known colloquially as a period for human females, with a cycle that lasts about 28 days) throughout the fertile years of women and for some time beyond.

The uterus is essential in sexual response by directing blood flow to the pelvis and to the external genitalia, including the ovaries, vagina, labia, and clitoris. The uterus is needed for uterine contractions to occur during a woman's orgasm.

The Fallopian Tubes

Connected to the uterus are the two fallopian tubes extending laterally for about four inches in opposite directions. This is where the human ovum (egg) and sperm cells come together and fertilization occurs. The fallopian tubes transport the ovum from the ovaries to the uterus, but the tubes do not make direct contact with the ovaries. The fallopian tubes have little finger-shaped projections, called fimbriae, at the ends, which sweep the egg into the fallopian tube.

The fallopian tubes are severed when a woman is sterilized. The medical process is called a tubal ligation. The woman is put under a general anesthesia for this procedure, performed in a surgical setting. It is seen as permanent, but it can be reversed through extensive microsurgery.

One last key point regarding the fallopian tubes is that they are very sensitive to infection, and when infections occur, they leave scar tissue that blocks the natural progression of the fertilized egg to the uterus. When this occurs, the fetus starts to develop in the tube until it ruptures the tube. This can be a life-threatening medical emergency for a woman.

The more a woman smokes, the higher her risk of an ectopic pregnancy. Pelvic inflammatory disease (PID) is often the result of an infection caused by sexually transmitted diseases such as chlamydia or gonorrhea.

Endometriosis, which can cause scar tissue to form in or around the fallopian tubes, can also lead to the problem. Exposure to the chemical Diethylstilbestrol (DES) before a female is born can also lead to PID. DES is a synthetic estrogen that was developed to supplement a woman's natural estrogen production.

The Ovaries

The ovaries are a pair of almond-sized organs that are attached by ligaments on both sides of the uterus. They have two very important functions that affect a woman's sexuality. One is that they produce the sex hormones estrogen and progesterone. The ovaries also hold the human eggs (ova). When a baby girl is born, she already has about 1,000,000 ovarian follicles. Each ovarian follicle contains a hollow ball of cells with an immature egg in the center. During childhood, the body absorbs approximately half of these ovarian follicles. By the time a girl reaches puberty and her menstrual cycle begins, only about 400,000 ovarian follicles are left to develop into mature eggs. Only 400 of those eggs are released in a woman's lifetime. If you ever consider being an egg donor, you will see that you have many to spare.

The Male External Sexual Anatomy

Unlike the female external sexual organs, the male external sexual organs are talked about, but they are not out there on display in magazines and books. In movies, women's bodies are revealed, but it's a rare occurrence to see a man's penis. Once in a while, a man's rear end is shown, but that's about it. This has all changed with the advent and accessibility of the Internet. By viewing pornography sites, teens and adults have easy access to the sexual anatomy of both sexes in detail. The problem with information obtained on the Internet is that immature or uninformed individuals can't tell the difference between what is fake and what is real. The mythology of sexual anatomy continues, and teens especially are misled with inaccurate information.

Where females find it difficult to view their genitalia, the male genitalia are easily visible. As a result, a man is very aware of the appearance of his own penis and scrotum. He may know what they look like and where they are located, but that doesn't mean he has a deeper understanding of how his genitals work, especially on a psychological level.

The Penis

There are many slang or street names used instead of the word penis. These labels connote a certain meaning and implication. Some of these names include: prick, dick, wanger, cock, pecker, dong, meat, member, hammer, joint, John Henry, and Johnson. What I find interesting is that some of these names have a dual meaning. This attitude reflects some type of psychological split when it comes to our acceptance of our genitals. When we call someone a prick or a dick in a derogatory tone, it shows that we feel some hostility toward our own genitals. I like my penis; it serves me very well, so why would I have contempt for its existence? Using the word dick or prick in a negative context seems conflicting.

Basically, the penis is a cylindrical organ with three columns of spongy tissue. Each of these columns is filled with small cavities that act just like sponges and are capable of temporarily storing blood. When a sponge is dry, its size is generally small, but when it comes into contact with water, it soaks up the water and increases in size. This is exactly what happens inside a penis, but instead of water being absorbed by the spongy bodies, it is blood that causes the spongy bodies to increase in size. This increase is what creates the physiological response of erection.

The penis has arteries and veins supplying blood to it, which allows it to function sexually. Arteries bring blood into the penis, and veins carry blood away from the penis. The penis can either be limp or erect, depending on the flow of blood. During sexual arousal, the arteries dilate, and more blood enters the penis than can leave because the veins leaving the penis constrict. Pressurized blood is trapped in the penis, and this blood causes the penis to elongate and stiffen. The penis is erect.

The penis has two functions. One is ejaculation, and the other is urination. Ejaculation is involved with the **secretion** of fluids from the seminal glands and the prostate, whereas urination

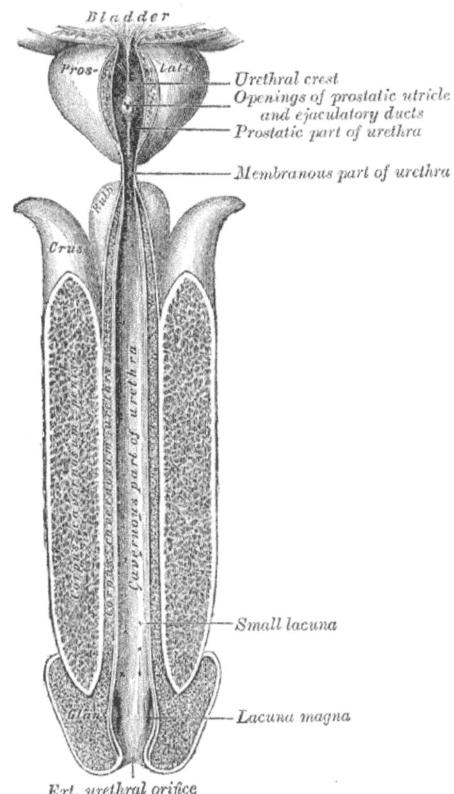

Figure 6: Male extrenal sex organs. Henry Gray, "Male extrenal sex organs," http://commons.wikimedia.org/wiki/File:Gray1142.png. Copyright in the Public Domain.

deals with the **excretion** of waste products, mainly urine from the bladder. There is a PC muscle at the root of the penis that aids in these two biological processes.

The actual shaft of the penis has relatively few nerve endings, especially in a fully erect state. In contrast, the glans or tip of the penis is well endowed with many nerve endings and is very sensitive to touch and stimulation.

The coronal ridge at the back edge of the glans is especially rich in nerve endings. Some men have the glans area of their penis covered with what is called the foreskin prepuce. This is a fold of skin which covers the glans, but it can be pulled back to expose the glans area. A large percentage of men in the United States have their foreskin removed at birth; this process is called circumcision.

The general reason for circumcision is for cleanliness. There are tiny glands behind the corona and foreskin that produce and secrete a cheese-like substance called smegma. Some believe that this material creates a good environment for bacteria to foster and grow. Others don't see any harmful effects of smegma, and, in fact, believe that it is beneficial to the glans of the penis. They use this argument to support their belief that circumcision is not necessary.

Today a debate exists about whether to perform a circumcision or not.

Some believe that a male is born with a prepuce covering the glans of his penis and there is no medical necessity to have it removed. Other believe that for health reasons it is beneficial to have an circumcision. Some believe that circumcision effects sexual responsiveness of the penis. Some say it enhances it, where others feel it limits sensitivity. Masters and Johnson in their research for that it didn't impact sensitivity either way.

Other reasons for circumcision are religious or cultural. For Jews, circumcision is a tradition where every Jewish boy has his foreskin removed after eight days of life, as prescribed in the Bible. In Islam, circumcision is mentioned in some writings, but not in the Koran. Some scholars state that circumcision is recommended, but others say that it is obligatory. While endorsing circumcision for males, Islamic scholars note that it is not a requirement for converting to Islam.

There are many myths associated with the penis. A common one has to do with the mystique surrounding its size. The same fixation American culture has about the size of a woman's breasts is shared by men about the size of their penis. Some studies have shown that men think that there is a correlation between the size of their penis and the degree of their masculinity.

The question is, how do boys learn about penis size in the first place? Their first visual sighting of a mature penis may be their father's or older brother's. This is usually a shock because when they make the comparison to their own penis, they will think that they are pretty small in size. Right from the beginning, they may begin to feel inadequate. Boys don't check out other boys' penises in school. When they are in the locker room after their gym class in middle school or even in high school, they don't go around looking at other boys' genitals. When boys use the urinal in the bathroom, they don't take a peek at the boy's penis in the urinal next to theirs. They make sure that they stare straight ahead when they are relieving themselves. All of this isolation regarding the appearance of other boys' penises has the effect of keeping most boys ignorant of normal penis size.

Without any frame of reference regarding penis size, young males are susceptible to being set up for feelings of inadequacy. When young male adolescents look at pornography on the Internet, they are again making comparisons between themselves and what they see on their computer screens. Producers of pornography tend to look for the anatomical freak when it comes to penis size. They look for the guy who is the exception to the average penis size. If the producers can't find the exception, they will use computer graphics to create a guy with a gigantic penis. Pornography is typically a male fantasy; it's not reality. The problem is that teenage boys who are naive and unaware believe what they see is real. Again, they are comparing themselves to something that isn't real and therefore will feel inadequate. Internet spammers prey on the ignorance of these boys or men by sending out e-mails that promise penis enlargement, with statements like: "Give her a couple more inches and she will never leave you for someone else." Of course, none of these products work, but insecure males buy these things thinking that they can be like the men they see in pornography.

If men only understood that the deeper they go in the vagina during intercourse, the fewer the number of nerve endings that exist, resulting in less pleasure for a woman. Those extra two inches aren't necessary on a biological level for a woman to experience pleasure through intercourse, although some women may be aroused by the idea of a large penis on a psychological level, similar to how some men are aroused by large breasts visually.

The average size of an unstimulated, flaccid penis is just under four inches in length and one inch in diameter. The average size of a penis in the erect state is about six inches in length and one and a half inches in diameter. When a male has a larger flaccid penis, it doesn't get larger than six inches when it becomes erect. A smaller flaccid penis becomes larger to roughly six inches at full erection. So penises don't start out the same size before being aroused, but end up the same at full erection.

There are several incorrect stories about penis size that still exist in popular folklore. One common myth is that you can tell a man's penis size by his skeletal structure. The fact is that there is no relationship between skeletal size and penis size. Another myth is that African Americans have larger penises than Caucasian men. There is no truth to this, just some men's insecurity about their own sexuality. One other myth I am aware of is that you can tell a man's penis size by the size of his nose or the size of his feet, but again, there is no basis for this.

About the only thing most penises have in common is that they are the wrong size and shape as far as their owners are concerned. "It's not much of an exaggeration to say that penises in fantasyland come in only three sizes: large, extra large, and so big you can't get them through the front door," says author and psychologist Bernie Zilbergeld.(9)

Male Internal Sexual Anatomy

Most men are well aware of their external sexual anatomy given its visibility, but their understanding of their internal anatomy and its functioning isn't fully appreciated. To this end, I want to explore the internal anatomical world, which may shed some light on what occurs and what anatomical parts play a role in sexual functioning.

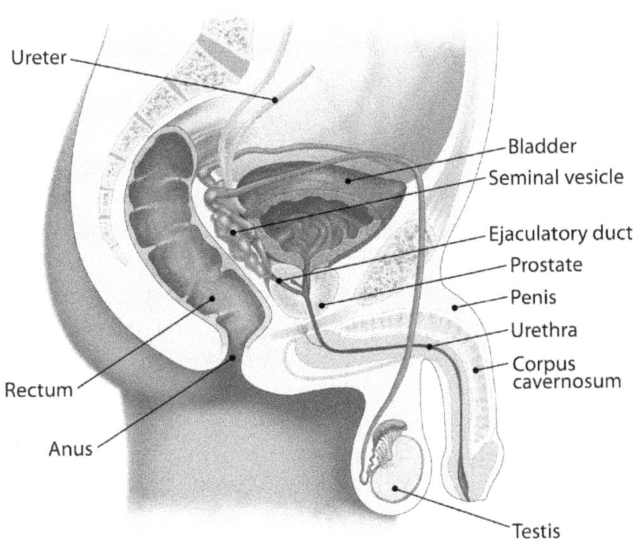

Figure 7: Male internal sex organs. Copyright © 2012 Depositphotos/kocakayaali.

The Testes

Many slang words exist for describing testicles, including balls, nuts, family jewels, and rocks. For our discussion, I will call them by their clinical term: testes or testicles.

The term testes comes from the Latin *testis*, which translates to witness. In biblical times, it was the custom when giving witness to hold the testicles of the person to whom one was making an oath, hence the modern word, testifying. The equivalent to this custom today would be to shake hands. Imagine how people would react if we reverted back to the biblical custom of testifying.

Testes are walnut-sized glands that vary in size, depending on the level of sexual arousal a male experiences. When a male becomes sexually aroused, blood tends to accumulate in the testes. This blood accumulation changes their color and sensitivity. It is also normal for the left testicle to hang lower than the right one in right-handed men, and the reverse for left-handed men.

The testes are very sensitive to pressure. Some men find gentle touching or squeezing of the scrotum to be sexually arousing. Others may wish to avoid this type of stimulation.

The testicles have two basic functions. One is to produce sperm cells, and the other is the production of the hormone testosterone. Within the testicles, sperm are produced in tightly coiled, microscopic seminiferous tubules. Billions of sperm are produced here each month. The hormone testosterone is produced in cells located near the seminiferous tubules.

One major concern about the testicles—other than cancer—is exposure to heat. The seminiferous tubules are very sensitive to heat, and too much can destroy them, rendering a male sterile or greatly reducing his sperm count. This can be a major issue if a male is trying to get his partner pregnant. You don't want to "cook the balls" when pregnancy is the goal. Stay away from hot spas or tight underwear. Mumps also used to be a major concern because it causes swelling of the testicles, which destroy the seminiferous tubules. With the advent of the mumps vaccine, the problem has been greatly reduced.

The Duct System

The male internal sexual anatomy is made up of tubes that transport sperm and other glandular fluids to be released outside a man's body. These tubes are called the duct system. Let's go on a journey with the sperm as they travel through the duct system and point out specific points of interest along the way.

After the sperm are produced in the tiny microscopic seminiferous tubules, they move into an area called the epididymis. The epididymis is made up of several hundred tubules that come together and form a tube in each testicle. This is the beginning of the duct system that transports the sperm to their destination. If the epididymis was uncoiled, it would measure 20 feet long. Once the sperm are produced, they spend from two to six weeks traveling through the epididymis, maturing and being reabsorbed by the body if they do not get the call to make the journey to be ejaculated out of their owner's body.

If the sperm do get the call to be ejaculated, they move from the epididymis to the second part of the duct system known as the vas deferens. There are two vasa deferentia (the plural form), one for each testicle. Each vas deferens is about 14 to 16 inches long. They transport sperm from the epididymis up and over the bladder to the ejaculatory duct. The vasa deferentia are surrounded by smooth muscle that contracts during ejaculation, helping the sperm move through the penis.

The vas deferens plays an important role in male sterilization. When a man decides he has does not want any more children, he might consider the medical procedure called a vasectomy.

The idea of having a vasectomy used to stir up a great deal of fear inside me. Hearing so many horror stories about the procedure and what happened afterward must have had a traumatic effect on my subconscious. When I actually had the procedure, I couldn't believe how little pain there was—and all the fears I had did not come to pass. The way the procedure is done today, there is virtually no discomfort. I was playing tennis the same day.

A vasectomy involves the surgeon putting a microscopic hole in the scrotum so he can access the vasa deferentia, cutting them and cauterizing the ends, attaching titanium clips to each end, and then reinserting the vasa deferentia back into the scrotum. There is no incision involved, and therefore no stitches.

A vasectomy is not something a man would undergo if he thinks he might change his mind down the road about having more children. The procedure can be surgically reversed, but it is very involved, and there is no guarantee. It's also very expensive.

The first point of interest along the sperm's journey through the duct system is the seminal vesicles. They look like two small sacs about two inches in length and are located behind the bladder. In the past, it was believed that they stored semen, which is how they got their name.

The seminal vesicles produce most of the content of semen (also called seminal fluid). About 70 percent of the seminal fluid in humans comes from the seminal vesicles. The seminal vesicles make most of the semen, but during ejaculation, most of the ejaculate has sperm, rather than semen in it. The use of seminal fluid is not known, since sperm do not move or survive well in semen. Some think that it acts as a fluid to stop sperm from another male impregnating the female so that the children of only one male can survive.

Seminal fluid contains proteins, enzymes, fructose, mucus, vitamin C, and flavins. The fructose gives sperm energy and "food" so they can continue their journey all the way to their destination. A tube connects the seminal vesicles to the ejaculatory duct so it is able to release the seminal fluid during ejaculation.

The next point of attraction along the sperm's journey through the duct system is the prostate gland. The function of the prostate is to store and secrete a slightly alkaline fluid, milky or white in appearance, that usually constitutes 20 to 30 percent of the volume of the semen along with sperm cells and seminal vesicle fluid. This prostatic fluid gives semen its characteristic odor.

The alkalinity of semen helps neutralize the acidity of the vaginal tract, prolonging the life span of sperm. The alkalization of semen is primarily accomplished through secretion from the seminal vesicles. The prostate also contains some smooth muscles that help expel semen during ejaculation.

The prostate becomes an issue for men over the age of 50, when it tends to become enlarged. The problem with the prostate growing in size is the impact this has on ducts traveling through the prostate, especially the urinary duct. It causes men with this problem to urinate more often or gives them the sense that they need to urinate.

In addition to the issue of developing an enlarged prostate is the concern over prostate cancer. It's important for men over 50 to have their prostate checked on a yearly basis. Early detection is critical to recovery and treatment.

The last gland or point of interest along the journey of the sperm is called the Cowper's gland. During sexual arousal, each gland produces a clear, viscous secretion known as pre-ejaculate. This fluid helps to lubricate the female urethra for sperm to pass through, neutralizing traces of acidic urine in the urethra, and helps flush out any residual urine or foreign matter. It is possible for this fluid to pick up sperm, remaining in the urethral bulb from previous ejaculations, and carry them out prior to the next ejaculation.

The mistake that many couples make is that they can practice the withdrawal method of birth control, thinking this will protect them from pregnancy. They believe they can withdraw the penis before ejaculation occurs and be safe from the possibility of pregnancy. This is not true. A man can get his lover pregnant because the Cowper's gland releases the tiny clear drops of fluid immediately prior to ejaculation, and he can't tell when this happens. The problem is that the pre-ejaculate may contain sperm cells from a previous ejaculation. There is some debate regarding the possibility of pregnancy, but why take the risk, unless you are comfortable with the possibility of becoming pregnant.

Excretion versus Secretion

The two terms, excretion and secretion, become confused in many people's minds and cause misconceptions regarding the biological fluids involved in sexual experiences. Semen, which is made up of fluids released from the seminal vesicles and the prostate gland, is considered a secretion and has nothing to with waste products. Excretions, on the other hand, are materials that are considered waste products, including urine, sweat, and fecal matter.

Vaginal fluids produced during sexual arousal are another example of secretions and don't fall into the category of waste products. The saliva in our mouth is a secretion and we don't consider it "dirty." Many people have a psychological aversion to sexual fluids because they make the mistake of seeing them as excretions and therefore offensive. This can inhibit the opportunity for oral sexual experiences, limiting a couple's overall sexual pleasure.

Works Cited

1. Chalker, Rebecca. The Clitoral Truth: The Secret World at Your Fingertips. New York: Seven Stores Press, 2000.
2. Yael, Tamir. Hands Off Clitoridectomy: What our revulsion reveals about ourselves. http://new.bostonreview.net/BR21.3/Tamir.html
3. http://health.howstuffworks.com/sexual-health/female-reproductive-system/hymen-dictionary1.htm
4. www.afraidtoask.com/tag/vulva/
5. http://www.greatsexafter40.com/
6. Ladas, A., Whipple, B., & Perry, J. *The G Spot and Other Discoveries About Human Sexuality* (Dell Publishing, 1982, reprint, 1983), 75.
7. http://womenshealth.about.com/cs/azhealthtopics/a/vagdouching.htm
8. http://womenshealth.about.com/cs/cevicalconditions/a/cervixwhatis.htm
9. Zilbergeld, Bernie. *The New Male Sexuality.* New York: Bantam Books, 1992.

5

Sexual Physiology

Now that we have looked at sexual anatomy, this chapter will discuss the subject of sexual physiology. Physiology addresses what happens on a biological level during the human sexual experience. This is the action part of sex. It's where the fun, excitement, and pleasure can happen. The subject of physiology may imply something clinical or boring. Far from it. For the most part, we will be exploring the question, "What creates a sexual response?"

Even though I am discussing a biological subject, I will concentrate on the psychological aspects and implications as much as possible. My academic background and clinical experience is in the area of psychology, not biology, so please take that into consideration.

Early Sex Researchers

Scientific or medical knowledge in the area of human sexual physiology is rather new when compared to our culture's understanding and knowledge of human physiology in general. The medical community didn't really start studying sexual physiology until midway through the 20th century. The first individual to shed a light on sexual physiology was Alfred Kinsey, along with his group of researchers. Kinsey was a biologist who founded the Institute for Sex Research at Indiana University in 1947. Kinsey's research on human sexuality laid the foundation for the modern field of human sexology.

Kinsey and his associates went around the world and interviewed men, and later women, about specific aspects of their sexual practices. Once the researchers finished their interviews, they compiled their data. This was the first time that any scientific approach was taken to find out firsthand what people actually did sexually. With their results, in 1948, Kinsey published his book, *Sexual Behavior in the Human Male*, which he followed up with in 1953 in another book, *Sexual Behavior in the Human Female*. Both books reached the top of the best-seller lists and turned Kinsey into an instant celebrity.

Perhaps his greatest contribution was to bring a long overdue ending to the dark ages on the subject of human sexuality, which opened the door for the work of William Masters and Virginia Johnson.

At Washington University in St. Louis, Missouri, Masters and Johnson did their pioneer research into the nature of human sexual response and behavior. William Masters, MD, was a gynecologist by training, and Virginia Johnson was his research assistant. In addition to studying the human sexual response, they also developed the diagnosis and treatment of disorders and sexual dysfunctions, which laid the foundation for the field of sexual therapy.

Masters and Johnson took the work of Kinsey to another level. Kinsey depended on case histories, interviews, and secondhand information. Masters and Johnson did their research under laboratory conditions, using technology to gather their information. This scientific approach had never been taken to study human sexual behavior.

Starting in 1956, William Masters hired Virginia Johnson to help in the interviewing and screening of volunteers. The study was conducted over an 11-year period, with 382 women and 312 men participating. The subjects ranged in age from 18 to 89 and were paid for their time. Masters and Johnson observed and recorded 14,000 sexual acts. They studied intercourse in many positions between happily married couples, couples with problems, and individuals, both heterosexual and homosexual.

After they did their research, they published two books that became best sellers and were translated into more than 30 languages. The first book, *The Human Sexual Response*, was released in 1966; their follow-up book, *Human Sexual Inadequacy*, was published in 1970. I owe a great deal of gratitude to Masters and Johnson because of their work, as it greatly influenced my professional career as a sex therapist and a college professor of human sexuality.

The Human Sexual Response

Most people who are not educated in the area of human sexuality believe that the human sexual response is just a simple process—a sexual stimulus is presented, and an individual responds. But it's not that one-dimensional. The human sexual response is made up multiple of components. When I meet with a patient who is not responding sexually, I need to explore all these components to find out where the difficulty may exist.

The first area that I need to check is whether any possible biological or medical issues might be involved in the patient's lack of sexual response. Usually, I want the patient to have a physical examination from their doctor to make sure that they are in good health. I wouldn't want to spend time exploring the psychological concerns when they may just need more testosterone, for example.

Once the patient has medical clearance, then I start looking at the psychological areas that influence a patien't sexual response. First, I explore with the patient their **emotions** in relation to their past or current sexual experiences. How do they feel about sex? Do they feel fear, anger, anxiety, or disgust, or do they feel joy and pleasure? Secondly, I explore their **thoughts** as they relate to sex in general or with their current relationship with their partner.

The next area I investigate is their **past** and what they have learned about sex in general from their childhood. What did the patient learn from their parents, their religious experience, their peers, or their education? All these influences can shape an individual's attitude toward sex, which can possibly inhibit their sexual response.

The last psychological component is the patient's **values** as they relate to sex. These values could either be on a personal level or from their culture. Where they grew up or what their ethnicity may be can have a direct effect on their sexual response.

You can see that there is nothing simple or one-dimensional about the human sexual response. It is rather complex and is made up of both psychological and medical components.

Sexual Arousal

When the average person talks about being sexually aroused, she may use terms like turned on, revved up, horny, super-hot, or excited. All these terms relate to some type of energy system. Sexual response is all about an activated state of sexual energy involving the sex organs and the nervous system. The organ that controls the nervous system is the brain. The brain is labeled the "sex organ" because of the role it plays in mediating an individual's sexual response.

A person can become sexually aroused on a cerebral level with no visible physical changes occurring in the body. Sexual arousal can be so intense that it can block out an individual's awareness of everything else going on around him. It can occur under a variety of circumstances and from many different sources.

Sexual excitement occurs in all age groups, from infants to the elderly. This doesn't mean that a child has the cognitive ability to identify or label their response as being sexual, but it nonetheless occurs on a physiological level. There is a general attitude that once a person reaches a certain age, they aren't capable of responding sexually because they are "over the hill." This is a myth; there is no cut-off age when an individual is no longer capable of sexual arousal. Their response may not be the same as when they were younger, but it's still possible, given they are in good health.

Sexual arousal can occur when a person is asleep as well as when she is awake. An interesting fact is that both men and women have automatic sexual arousal experiences during sleep that are independent of anything occurring sexually on a mental level. Men have about half a dozen erections during a night's sleep, each lasting about five to ten minutes. Women lubricate in a similar way. Sometimes, men wake up in the middle of one of these automatic erections and label it as a "piss hard-on" because they usually have to urinate at the same time, which is why they are awake.

The Two Main Physiological Reactions

Overall, two physiological effects occur in the body during sexual arousal. The first one is called **vasocongestion**, an increase of blood flow that becomes localized to specific body tissues. During sexual excitement, vasocongestion occurs in the male's penis to render it hard and erect. The equivalent occurrence in a woman is an increase in blood flow to the walls of her vagina, which, in turn, creates lubrication and the hardening of the clitoris. Another example of vasocongestion during sexual arousal is a "sex flush," where the increase of blood gives the chest the look of a red rash. In addition, vasocongestion causes hardening of the nipples in both men and women.

The Myth of "Blue Balls"

One example of vasocongestion that has been blown into a sexual myth is what men call "blue balls." Loosely translated, the idea is that the testicles turn blue during sexual excitement due to the increase of blood in this area. The myth is that a man will experience a great deal of suffering and pain if he doesn't experience ejaculation. This story has been used as a ploy to manipulate the man's partner to continue with the sexual experience, even though the partner may not want to carry on further. How could their partner leave them with so much pain and agony? Their partner may believe this to be real and continue with the sexual experience, even though they might want to stop. Although there may be a great deal of vasocongestion in the testicles and some discomfort with continued stimulation, if the stimulation stops, then all the blood drains back to a pre-arousal state, and the discomfort is resolved. In other words, what goes up comes down.

This same issue of vasocongestion to the pelvic area occurs for women. If they don't experience sexual resolution, they may experience an unpleasant pelvic "heaviness," but this condition is only temporary.

The second general physiological reaction during sexual response is called **neuromuscular tension**. This term refers to a buildup of energy and tension throughout the body's muscles and nervous system. This includes both flexing (which is voluntary) and contractions (which are involuntary). The most obvious examples of this are the muscle contractions that occur during both male and female orgasm. The muscle tension also causes facial grimaces and twitches in the hands and feet.(1) Usually, the term tension is viewed as something negative, but in the context of sexual arousal, it's a positive experience.

Benchmarking a Sexual Response or Experience

Many people are tempted to evaluate the quality of a sexual response by the size, speed, or intensity of an orgasm or an erection, or by the degree of vaginal lubrication. They use these determinants as a way to judge their proficiency as a lover. The degree to which one experience is "better" than another is a subjective determination. It all depends on the individual and how he evaluates the experience.

This entire evaluation process is problematic. The idea of judging what occurs during the sexual experience can lead to the problem of spectating, which will be discussed in detail in the chapter on sexual dysfunctions.

A tendency I have observed with many couples is that they tend to "benchmark" what their sexual experience was like for them. For example, let's take a couple who has been dating for a while and has been putting off having sex until they know one another on a more intimate level. The big moment finally arrives, and they have this incredible sexual experience. They give it a ten on their rating scale of one to ten, with ten being the best score you can get.

The mistake they make is that the next time they have sex together they compare their sexual activity to their "benchmark experience." Their last experience may only be an eight compared to their benchmark, which devalues the experience. A better approach is to stop judging and comparing sexual experiences and just enjoy them. When judgment invades any sexual experience, it will inhibit the level of pleasure an individual will experience. Instead, look at each sexual experience as unique and different, not that one is better than another. If you keep eating gourmet food every night, even that will become boring.

The Four Stages of the Human Sexual Response Cycle

Even though there are differences between the way men and women respond sexually, Masters and Johnson discovered that men and women pass through four basic stages during the sexual response cycle. These four stages, or phases, that blend into one another are: excitement, plateau, orgasm, and resolution.

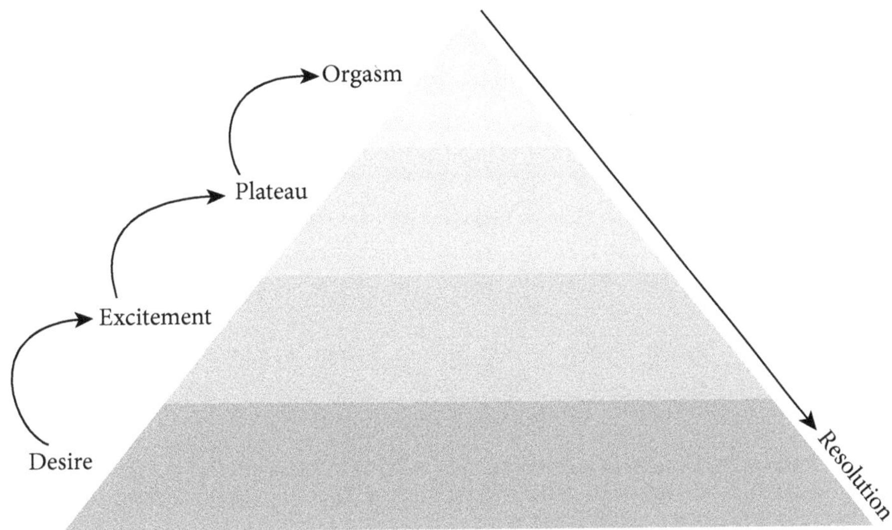

Figure 8: Sexual response cycle.

There is a wide variety of individual variation in the duration and intensity of these stages. The perception of excitement and response varies for any given individual and the type of stimulation: oral, manual, penile, or vibrator.

On a broader level, men typically go through the response cycle with greater uniformity. They enter the excitement phase rapidly and then move on to the plateau stage, where they don't spend much time, then move into the orgasmic phase by ejaculating, ending up at the resolution phase.

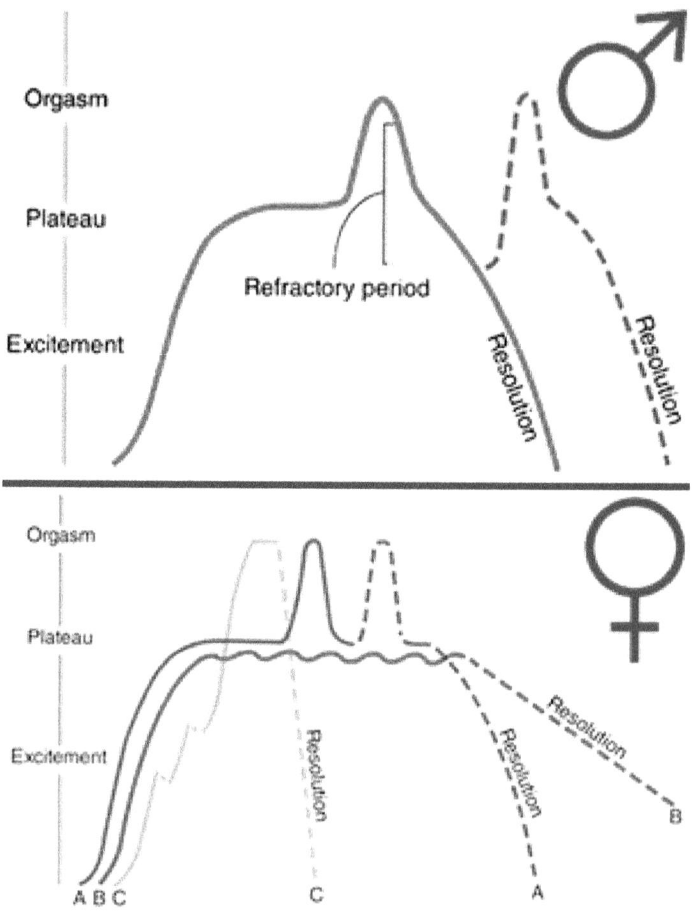

Figure 9: Sexual response cycle graph. Avril1975, "Sexual response cycle graph," http://commons.wikimedia.org/wiki/File:Sexual-response-cycle.png. Copyright in the Public Domain.

On the other hand, a woman's path through the phases of the sexual response cycle is much more varied when compared to men. A woman can get excited and move into a plateau phase and stay there for a while, and then go back down to excitement and then back to plateau, have an orgasm and back to plateau, and then experience another orgasm, and then go to resolution. Women don't necessarily follow the same pattern from one sexual experience to another.

Physiological Changes and Events During Each Phase

Excitement

The excitement phase is the first phase of the sexual response cycle. Like all phases of the sexual response, it varies from person to person and situation to situation: It can last anywhere from less than a minute to over several hours. It includes neuromuscular tension and increased heart rate and blood pressure. Also, many sexual areas can become engorged with blood, including the clitoris, breasts, penis, and testes. The sexual organs often gain a deeper color in this phase as well. A sex flush, which is a pink or red rash on the chest or breasts, can occur in both men and women, though it is more common in women. During the excitement phase, a man's penis becomes erect, though the erection is not necessarily completely hard-it can vary between unaroused, partially aroused, and fully aroused states.

The testes also elevate and engorge with blood. In women, the clitoral shaft gets bigger, the labia majora separate, and the labia minora enlarge, while often becoming darker. Also, some women produce considerable amounts of lubrication at this point, though others only produce a small amount.

Plateau

In the plateau phase, sexual tension continues to grow as a precursor to orgasm. This phase can be very brief, from two seconds to a few minutes. Many people find that extending the length of the plateau period can lead to more intense orgasms. This phase does not have a clear starting point, in which a person obviously shifts from excitement to plateau. In the plateau phase, everything that happened in the excitement phase continues, and it becomes more prominent. Heart and breathing rates continue to rise, muscle tension increases, and sex flushes and genital coloration become more noticeable. During the plateau phase for women, the outer one-third of the vagina becomes especially engorged with blood, creating a structure called the orgasmic platform.

Note that the word plateau is usually used to describe a leveling-off, where there are no real changes. In these stages, however, the plateau is not a static, boring place. Very powerful surges of sexual tension or pleasure occur in this stage; for example, both men and women often experience faster heart and breathing rates.

Orgasm

Orgasm is the shortest phase of the sexual response cycle, typically lasting only several seconds. Women can have a slightly longer orgasm than men. While men almost always experience orgasm after the plateau phase, many women can experience the plateau stage without reaching orgasm. Usually, men experience orgasm and ejaculation in conjunction with each other, but ejaculation does not always occur at the time of orgasm. Before ejaculation can occur, the seminal fluids gather in the ejaculatory ducts and upper urethra. This produces a feeling that orgasm is inevitable. Then, the semen is expelled out of the penis at the time of orgasm. When a woman orgasms, the uterus and orgasmic platform contract in rhythmic waves of muscular movement.

It is interesting to note that orgasms do not seem to differ by gender; that is, men and women feel quite similar things during orgasm. In one study, college students provided descriptions of orgasm. Researchers compared the descriptions using a standard psychological rating scale, and found no distinguishable differences between men's and women's descriptions. Both males and females tended to describe orgasm with words such as "waves of pleasure in my body," corresponding to the rhythmic muscle contractions that occur during orgasm.

Resolution

In this phase, the body returns to its original, unexcited state. Some of the changes occur rapidly, whereas others take more time. The resolution phase begins immediately after orgasm if there is no additional stimulation.(2)

So far, we have discussed the Masters and Johnson model of sexual response. Helen Singer Kaplan, a sex therapist, modified the Masters and Johnson sexual response cycle based on her work treating sexual dysfunction problems in men and women. Her model, which she developed in the 1970s, is called the triphasic model of human sexual response.

Dr. Kaplan added a prior stage of sexual desire while eliminating the resolution phase that she believes to be an absence of sexual response, rather than part of the cycle itself. In addition, Kaplan eliminated the plateau phase as defined by Masters and Johnson because she believed that it is essentially a continuation of the excitement phase and because it is of little value in sex therapy, due to the virtual impossibility of a patient distinguishing it from the excitement phase. Therefore, her model has only three phases: sexual desire, excitement, and orgasm.(3)

The Two Major Physiological Differences Between Men and Women

The first major physiological difference is that men experience something called a **refractory period** as a part of the sexual response cycle. This is the time between one orgasm and another. Most men are unable to maintain or achieve an erection during this time, and many perceive a psychological feeling of satiation and are temporarily uninterested in further sexual activity. The penis may be hypersensitive, and further sexual stimulation may even feel painful during this time frame.

How long the refractory period lasts varies with the age of the individual, nutrition, and overall health. The actual time frame can be minutes to days. According to some studies, 18-year-old males have a refractory period of about 15 minutes, while those in their 70s take about 20 hours, with the average for all men being about half an hour.(4) Unlike most men, most women do not experience a refractory period immediately after orgasm and in many cases are capable of attaining additional, multiple orgasms through further stimulation.(5) The female sexual response is more varied than that of men; many women experience clitoral hypersensitivity after orgasm, which effectively creates a refractory period. These women may be capable of further orgasms, but the pain involved in getting there makes the prospect undesirable.(6)

The other important physiological difference between men and women is something called **ejaculatory inevitability**. Once a male reaches a certain level of arousal and moves from the plateau stage to the orgasmic stage and emission occurs, it's almost impossible for a man to stop the ejaculatory process. Some women, on the other hand, can reach very high levels of arousal during the plateau stage and cannot—for many different psychological reasons—experience an orgasm. This can lead to a great deal of frustration and disappointment for women who experience this difficulty.

The Psychological Significance of the Plateau Stage of the Sexual Response Cycle

It is my belief that the plateau stage of the sexual response cycle holds a great deal of psychological significance for both men and women. I especially want to look at how understanding the psychology of this stage is important for men in general.

The plateau stage represents two major factors that most people don't recognize. The first factor is that when a person is involved in the plateau stage of the sexual response cycle, he is potentially experiencing an incredible level of sexual pleasure. I can't think of any experience that is so full of pleasure. The plateau stage is where the most sustained sexual pleasure is experienced during the sexual response. This stage provides the greatest opportunity for prolonged sexual pleasure. I compare this experience to eating the most decadent dessert in an expensive French restaurant, where you want to savor every bite of sweet pleasure. You just don't want the pleasure to end. Experiencing an orgasm is awesome, but how long does it actually last? On average, only 18 to 20 seconds. Those are fantastic seconds, but the experience doesn't last very long, especially for males, because they can't have another orgasm. That's it—the fun and pleasure is over—compared to women, who have the potential of having more orgasms for continued sexual pleasure.

You might ask, "What's the issue with a lot of sexual pleasure?" The psychological issue involves men and their relationship with pleasure in general and sexual pleasure specifically. When I ask men what they do for pleasure, their response usually involves some form of work. They respond with answers such as: "I work around my house," "I work out in the gym," or "I work on my car." Their concept of pleasure is some type of goal-oriented pursuit, where they are doing some type of activity. The one big exception is the couch potato, who watches television for pleasure—but this habit is often tinged with guilt because this really isn't considered an acceptable activity.

Males in our culture are taught from an early age through various psychological message delivery systems that a man must always be accomplishing something. He must produce, achieve, and produce something worthwhile and tangible for his time spent. Otherwise, his time is wasted. As Bernie Zilbergeld states in his book, *Male Sexuality*, the three A's of manhood are achieve, achieve, and achieve.(7)

Being brought up with the same programing made it difficult for me to just sit on the beach and enjoy the experience through all my senses. I couldn't just sit on the beach, because I had all these voices in my head saying, "Dan, you are wasting your time sitting here. You are not accomplishing anything." These voices made it very difficult for me to **relax** and just share the time with my girlfriend, and later my wife.

If I was at a beach that had waves where I could body surf, I was comfortable because then I could do some type of activity and I wasn't bored just sitting there. Was I being intimate with my wife when I was out in the water body surfing? Not really, because she wasn't comfortable being out there in the water with me. I was out in the water, and she sat on the beach. And as a result, we weren't intimately involved, assuming that was the intent of the experience.

The common psychological programming that males are given in this culture is that we don't have permission to enjoy pleasure for its own sake; we are taught to work, accomplish, achieve, and produce. This belief blocks our ability to just stay and enjoy the plateau stage of sexual arousal. We need to be striving toward a goal—otherwise, we are wasting our time. In order to enjoy sexual pleasure, you need to be in the moment and just "hang out" with the pleasure. So, it can be difficult for a man to stay at the plateau stage without an attitude shift occurring.

Besides being the most pleasurable part of the human sexual response, the plateau stage also has psychological significance—it represents the most potentially intimate position you can experience with your lover. Both partners are naked, vulnerable, and open to each other while experiencing a very high level of sexual arousal. To sustain this level of physical vulnerability and sexual pleasure over time, an individual must be comfortable with being incredibly intimate with their lover.

For men in general, the actual experience of intimacy can also be difficult psychologically. They are just not comfortable with extended periods of physical intimacy. They just want to have sex, as opposed to making love for an extended period. They may talk about wanting this type of experience, but the reality is another story.

A major consequence of a man's inability to relax and enjoy the pleasure and intimacy of the plateau stage is that he really doesn't experience true sexual fulfillment on a deeper physical and emotional level. It tends to leave them wanting more sexual activity because when they have the opportunity for emotional and sexual satisfaction, they just want to move through it and go on to some other activity. This can leave men with "sexual malnutrition," as though they can never get enough sex. They live with a sex life that's like always eating fast food, providing quick relief for hunger, but with no real quality or substance.

I don't want to imply that only men have trouble with the plateau stage, because some women may not want to sustain it either. Their reasons are often different from those of men—they are generally more comfortable with intimacy—but if they don't feel emotionally close because of the lack of intimate communication in general with their lover, they won't want to sustain physical closeness.

If a woman isn't experiencing sexual pleasure during her sexual experience, she won't want to sustain the plateau stage, either. She may just want the whole experience to reach its conclusion in the quickest time possible.

Open yourself to the potential of the plateau stage and all its potential for pleasure and intimacy because it can last a long time. An orgasm is great, but it's over pretty quickly.

Sexual Adequacy in America

In 1973, when I was training as a sex therapist, I came across an article by Philip Slater called, "Sexual Adequacy in America"(8), which describes how an individual's sexual adequacy is judged physiologically. Slater observes an inequality between how men and women are judged. A double standard exists. I think this still holds true today.

A male is judged sexually adequate if he is able to produce an **erection**. Without the ability to perform sexually with a hard erection, a male judges himself (and is judged by others) as being sexually inadequate. A woman is judged sexually adequate if she is able to achieve an **orgasm**.

In addition to these two criteria, a man is defined as adequate if he is able to bring his female partner to orgasm with his penis. A woman is defined as adequate if she is able to achieve an orgasm rapidly through penile penetration/intercourse.

Looking at these definitions of sexual adequacy, a man is good if he can delay orgasm, whereas a woman is good if she can accelerate her orgasmic response. Because of these judgments, a double standard exists between men and women when it comes to determining sexual adequacy.

Slater believes that when examining these definitions of sexual adequacy from the standpoint of the ability to tolerate and sustain sexual pleasure without release: **the fact is that women can**

absorb and tolerate more sexual pleasure than men. It was always thought that males have a greater sexual capacity than females. The reverse is true. From the viewpoint of physical capacity or capability, women have an almost unlimited orgasmic potential when compared to men.

I believe this to be true as well. One of the major sexual myths that have been perpetrated on women over the years is that they take a long time to sexually respond to stimulation. They were judged inadequate because they compared their sexual response rate to their male partners. Before the 1970s and the women's liberation movement, sexual fulfillment was meant to be for men, so it was all about them. This is a classic example where male sexuality is used as the benchmark for what is sexually adequate, for both men and women.

Why is being in a hurry sexually a good thing? Men talk about wanting to be sexual all the time—at least that's the stereotype. They make a big deal about having sex, but when the opportunity arrives, they seem to be in a big hurry to get the sexual act over. If their partner isn't in a hurry as well, they put her down for taking so long. How many times do I hear women express their dissatisfaction with their sex life because there isn't much time spent on foreplay?

Women in this culture are allowed to experience pleasure in general. They don't question their gender or their sexual orientation, unlike men. A woman can create a pleasurable experience by taking a long, hot bath with scented candles, soft lights, and a glass of wine, and just relax and enjoy the self-soothing experience. What do men do? They just jump in the shower, in and out, and that's it, on to the next thing. They might sit in a spa, but that has the agenda of sex involved. Men can learn to experience pleasure—they just have to let go of the goal of going somewhere else.

Slater also makes the point that work and sexual pleasure are natural enemies, and the more personal the commitment to work, the more inroads it makes into one's sexual life. This has been one of the major reasons why the lack of sexual desire and frequency has become the number one sexual problem for couples today.

More Sexual Physiological Myths

The notion that all orgasms are intense, earth-shattering, explosive events is another widespread sexual misconception. This myth has resulted both from popular literature and from images of explicit sex on the Internet. It's common for popular writers to embellish their descriptions of female orgasms so that the uninformed fall prey to believing the author's fictional fantasy as reality. The same can be said for Internet pornography. Porn is acting—it isn't real, but developing adolescents may think that what they see is real, and then expect what they saw to be true in real life. They are setting themselves up for disappointment, and this will create many issues for future mental health professionals to deal with.

In pornography, a woman's orgasmic response is acted out to fit a man's fantasy. These males are going to be disappointed when they find out the reality when they are in an adult sexual relationship. They will probably try to make their female partner feel inadequate because she isn't living up to their false expectations.

How a woman experiences an orgasm during the sexual response cycle is her own experience. There is no right or wrong way to have an orgasm. Whatever way she has the experience of orgasm is great. There is no benchmarking one orgasmic experience and comparing all the orgasms that follow in some rating process to measure the degree of pleasure. For example, one time she might be loud and scream, and the next time she might be silent, but spasm a great deal. Both experiences may be very pleasurable, but very different. It's fine to enjoy the difference.

Another old myth is that a couple has to have mutual orgasms. They both need to come at the same time. If this happens, it can be an exhilarating and highly pleasurable experience. Where it becomes a problem is when the couple becomes so involved with the goal of both reaching orgasm at the same time that each of them is so focused on their partner's sexual response that they aren't enjoying their own experience. If mutual orgasms happen, that's great, but to work at trying to make this happen every time is too rigid and predictable.

The Male Sexual Response

Erection

For most of his lifetime, the healthy, normal man can physically lose and regain his erection several times during his sexual experience. There is nothing physically that prevents this from occurring, unless he has some type of medical condition such as prostate cancer.

The problem with gaining and losing erections is usually not a physical issue, but more a psychological problem. It's a man's emotional reaction to the loss of his erection. He gets angry, embarrassed, and anxious at the same time. These emotions don't foster any erotic feelings. They do not allow him to become aroused and respond with another erection once he loses his erection.

An erection is a vascular phenomenon that is triggered by a nervous system reflex. An erection is an involuntary response, which means that it happens automatically and doesn't require a decision by the brain. At the same time, the brain can also shut down the response.

Ejaculation

Under normal conditions of sexual excitement and with an erection, a male is able to follow these events with an ejaculation. The two components of the male sexual response, erection and ejaculation, are independent of each other. An ejaculation can happen in the absence of an erection, and vice versa. A male can ejaculate through mental fantasy in the absence of penile stimulation and feeling the emotion of anxiety and fear can inhibit ejaculation, even with adequate sexual stimulation occurring.

The Channels of Sexual Arousal and Response

If the brain is the real sex organ, how does the brain receive information that creates the sexual turn-on? What we call the sexual response is a process of considerable complexity. It's never completely automatic, even among those who are very sexually experienced. Decisions are made that allow us to respond to the stimulation we receive. There is no automatic connection for a man, for example, between touching a woman's breasts and the blood flow into his genitals. Many men think that there should be an automatic response, but that's not the way it really happens.

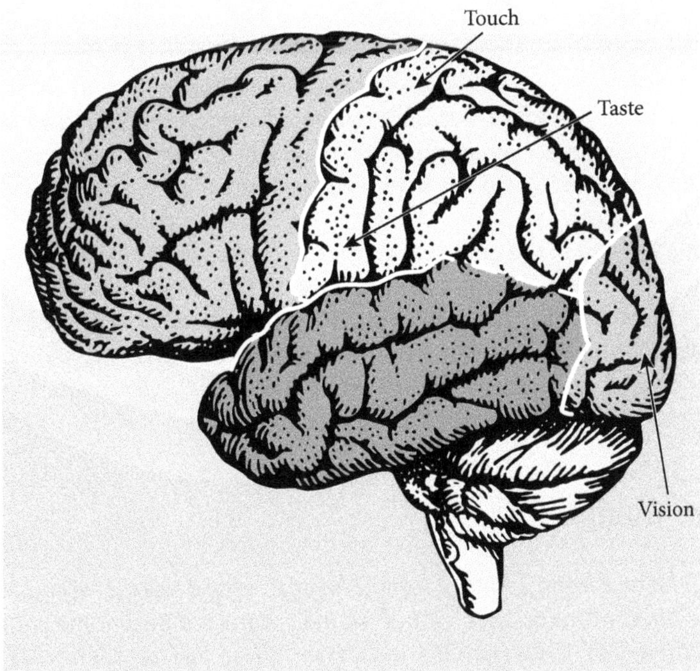

Figure 10: Sensory system and the brain. Copyright © 2011 Depositphotos/ Den.Barbulat.

Our senses provide us with the information that **we** define as being sexual. Our senses are the inputs to the brain; they provide us with the information that gives us the potential to create sexual arousal.

The Sense of Sight

Visual stimulation is a major sense that plays a key role in sexual arousal. This is especially true in American culture. For males, our first sexual focus is on what we see. We learn early in childhood to look at girls in sexual terms. It is almost a way to bond with other males to compare mental notes about the way girls look. When I was growing up, there was a special emphasis on female breasts. I think this is still true today. Everything was visual for males. If we didn't have real girls to stare at, then we would try to get hold of our father's *Playboy* magazine and look at the images. Today, the ability to look at images has gone way beyond anything in *Playboy* with the accessibility to the Internet and the availability of explicit images of naked women that make these magazines seem tame in comparison.

The problem with the heavy emphasis on visual stimulation is that what many men—especially developing male adolescents—don't realize is that many, if not most, of these images of female bodies are not real. All the outlets of the mass media manufacture these images using digital manipulation; they create a female image of perfection that truly doesn't exist in the real world.

When we stare at these images and they become etched on our brains, we forget and don't think at the time that these are false images.

The problem occurs when we look at our female lovers' bodies, and all we see are the imperfections, especially as we age. This leads to frustration, disappointment, and anger directed at our partners, and this reaction is an impediment to having a great sexual relationship. Of course, this judgment from their male partners has a very adverse effect on women, in terms of their own self-esteem and body image.

It was generally thought in the past that women did not respond sexually to visual stimulation in the same way as men do. I personally never thought that women checked men out sexually on a visual level. How wrong I was with this assumption. Women were observing visually, but because of social conditioning, just didn't talk about their reactions like men do. As I got older, I heard women talk about how other men looked all the time. *Playgirl* magazine displays sexual images of males just like its counterparts, *Penthouse* and *Playboy*.

The Sense of Sound

In the animal kingdom, certain auditory stimulation can provide sexual stimulation. Ducks have mating calls and different birds have certain sounds that send sexual messages that the time is right for sex to happen. Every spring, I hear male doves making their familiar call, sending the message to any female that is flying around in the neighborhood that his nest is set up for reproduction. I thought it was the other way around, but that is not the case.

Humans do not give each other vocalized sexual signals before performing a particular sexual activity. That is not to say that humans don't become sexually aroused by auditory stimulation. Certain auditory stimulation can cause sexual arousal. The sound of a couple making love in an adjacent room in a motel room may be erotic to some people. The sound of heavy breathing, or a woman screaming during the sex act may also be arousing to some.

Hearing erotic tapes that include explicit sex—not romance—can create sexual arousal in men and women. The assumption that women react only to the romantic tapes or at least that they prefer eroticism that is tempered with romance rather than straight-out sex is incorrect.

The Sense of Smell

The sense of smell is an important part of the initiatory stages of sexuality among our nearest animal relatives. "Across the animal world, creatures from insects to mammals release and receive sexual pheromones—scent hormones—signaling to the opposite sex that they're 'in the mood.' Males will travel miles, following the scent trail of a female. A female who wouldn't have given the time of day to some guy will suddenly find him very attractive. In fact, all she can think about is having his babies—and it all began with a whiff and a little chemistry."(8)

Are pheromones, human sex scents in humans, a myth, or are they real? At this point, it is difficult to give a definitive answer. "David Wolfgang-Kimball, a physiological researcher at the University of California at San Francisco proposed a new way of looking at pheromones, specifically in humans. With our highly developed intellect and rich complement of emotions, ambitions, motivations and desires, it may not be profitable to look at human pheromones the same way we look at animal pheromones. Instead of looking for odorants that cause a definite physiological response, it may behoove us to look at how possible pheromones affect our attitudes. We are not machines that blindly fall into some stereotyped behavior in response to an odor, but we may be machines that are nudged towards a type of behaviour by pheromones in concert with our higher intellect."(9)

If humans have pheromones like our relatives in the animal kingdom, we take care of them by removing their existence from our bodies. We Americans in particular are obsessed with ridding our bodies of any natural odors. We find their smell disgusting and definitely not erotic in any way. We take showers daily to wash away any odors. When we aren't in the shower, we use deodorants to make sure we don't give off any body scents. If we lived in a time when bathing was not so accessible or routine, we might have a different opinion and experience.

Today, we believe that we can replace our natural pheromones with artificial scents such as colognes and perfumes that we can purchase in our local department store or online. Americans and Europeans spend 12 billion dollars a year on perfume.(10) That's a lot of money to smell sexy.

Do perfume and cologne create sexual arousal physiologically in humans? The answer is no. The effect they provide is a conditioned stimulus that might create a sexual response, but this response is through learned conditioning, not physiology. The physiological response occurs after the fact that the conditioned stimulus is present; i.e., the perfume.

In other words, Jack might have numerous fantastic sexual experiences with Karen. Every time Jack has sex with Karen, she wears a particular perfume—let's say Chanel Coco Mademoiselle. Jack creates an association between the smell of the perfume and the experience of having great sex with Karen. Just the smell of that fragrance can get Jack sexually aroused to the possibility of have a great sexual experience. This is called a conditioned response.

In this case, the conditioned response would be considered positive, but negative conditioning can also occur. What if Karen cheats on Jack and he finds her in bed with another man? Now, if he smells that particular fragrance, he feels the pain associated with that triggered memory, as opposed to the pleasure of the past. If he dates a new woman and she wears the same fragrance, he will experience the pain again, and that could get in the way of him sexually responding to the new opportunity.

The Sense of Taste

Of the five senses, I used to think that taste was the least important in terms of influencing sexual arousal. I was pleased to learn that I was wrong. On the contrary, each person's skin has a particular taste that is perceived through kissing and contact of the tongue, and the special taste can produce strong sexual response. Some people report that the taste of certain foods can have an aphrodisiac effect on sexual arousal as well.

In an article called "Sex and the Five Senses," James R. Coffey writes that while it's true that our sense of taste is actually an extension of our ability to smell (taste is greatly limited when we can't smell), most men and women consider the mouth unsurpassed as a pleasure center. In fact, while a majority of women rate orgasm as the mark of an ultimate sexual encounter, they rate kissing as the most stimulating aspect overall. And while some men and women only symbolically caress their lover's body, others prefer to *taste* them—especially their lips, breasts, and sex organs. And since nibbling, licking, and sucking the breasts, ears, neck, and navel (and sometimes buttocks) are considered common foreplay for some, tasting automatically becomes a part of it. The various tastes of their lover's body become pleasurable triggers for sexual interest. Why, then, do we not routinely set out to incorporate our sense of taste into lovemaking? Why do we limit where and when we taste? Is it because social convention dictates that oral stimulation is depraved and perverted?(11)

The Sense of Touch

Of all the five senses, touch is the one that Americans don't pay enough attention to in their daily routines, especially within a sexual context. When we are babies and young children, we are held, cuddled, and caressed. We receive a great deal of tactile stimulation. Tactile stimulation is critical to a child's healthy development. Why is it as we move into adulthood that we experience less and less touch in our lives? Often, the only time any adult gets any touching is within a sexual context. This is especially true for males. Some believe that men want to have sex just to be touched; it's not just that they are so turned on. They confuse the need for touching with the need for sex. There might be a lot less violence if males got a lot more touching in their lives.

The perception of touch is mediated through nerve endings in the skin and deeper tissue. These nerve endings are distributed unevenly throughout the body. Before I trained as a sex therapist, I used to believe that the body had specialized sexual nerve endings that sent sexual messages to a part of the brain that would somehow cause sexual arousal. In addition, I thought that these sexual nerve endings were located in very specific parts of the body, like the penis or the vagina. I was later told that these areas were called the erogenous zones. More specifically, these zones were the breasts and the genital area. I have seen this diagrammed in old human sexuality textbooks.

It doesn't surprise me that over the years of listening to how couples describe the way they touch each other when they are sexually involved, they usually report that most of their touching activity went directly to the breasts and each other's genitals, in an attempt to arouse each other to have intercourse. They believed that these areas were the key areas to create arousal quickly, so that they could move directly to have sex.

As I became educated in human sexuality, I soon learned that on a physiological level, there isn't a "sexual nerve ending." The nerve endings located in my genitals are the same nerve endings located in my feet, hands, or neck. We have nerve endings all over our bodies. They may not be as concentrated as in the genitals such as the clitoris, but there are enough in the hands or feet to transmit pleasure to an individual's brain. As a teenager, I can still can remember how good it felt to hold a girl's hand as I walked her home, which was a very sexual experience at that time of my development.

When I understood the anatomical fact that there isn't a specialized sexual nerve ending, this changed my belief about the concept of the body's erogenous zones. The fact is that the whole body is potentially an erogenous zone because we have nerve endings all over our bodies. When these nerve endings are stimulated within an erotic context, our brains receive so much pleasure from all these nerve endings. It's just an incredible sexual experience.

A 5.1 Surround Sound Sexual Experience

Before there was 5.1 surround sound music reproduction, there was something called monaural sound, or "mono." There was just one speaker, one channel of sound being reproduced on a record player back in the day. Then, in the 1960s, stereo sound came out, which was a major development in sound reproduction. Now, we have five and six channels of sound in our family rooms that we use to listen to music or watch movies. Going back to monaural sound would be a shock to our collective auditory system.

I use this metaphor of sound reproduction to describe the way many couples today experience sex within their relationship. What is missing is the full range or spectrum of sensual pleasure. For many couples, they generally focus on one or maybe two of their senses. Generally, these include the sense of vision and sound. As I said earlier, the senses are the way that our brain receives information from our experience. The brain then may or may not apply a sexual meaning to this information; it just depends on the context of the situation. The brain is the ultimate sex organ, and the more sensual stimulation it receives, the greater the opportunity for sexual pleasure.

What I suggest to couples in order to improve their sexual experience is to take it from a mono experience to a 5.1 surround sound sensual feast. The way to enhance the experience is to turn up the volume on all the senses. Most people, especially men, focus on the visual aspect of sex and that's all. Not that there is anything wrong with this—it's just limiting. But what if we add some relaxing background music for a little auditory stimulation, along with some nice-smelling aromatherapy candles? Candles also do wonders for the visual ambience, as opposed to normal lighting. Perhaps add a nice glass of wine and chocolate-dipped strawberries, and top it off with a nice full-body massage to bring more touching to the experience. Now you have a surround sound 5.1 sexual experience that is loaded with sensuality. With all the senses operating, the level of pleasure associated with the sexual experience is increased. When sex and sensuality are mixed, the experience is incredible. Enjoy.

Recognizing Your Dominant Sense to Become a Better Lover

In the 1980s, I attended a weekend workshop with two individuals, Richard Bandler and John Ginder, from the University of California at Santa Cruz. They had studied the language that some famous family therapists used in their therapy sessions. One of their discoveries was that it was important to understand what the dominant sense was that the patient used to take in information from their outside world. If a patient's dominant sense was vision, they then would ask them a question like, "How does it *look* to you get married?" If the patient's dominant sense was auditory, they would say, "How does it sound to you get married?" I soon realized that my dominant sense at that time was vision. When I watch the video replay of my interviews on television, I notice that when the interviewer asks me a question, I always look up to the left, as if there was a monitor there with the answer. I was visualizing the response.

I understood this concept of dominant sense in general communication styles, but I didn't understand its relevance to sexual interaction and communication within the sexual context. When it came to my dominant sense in those days, it was the perception of touch.

One night, my lover at the time asked me if what she was doing to me sexually was pleasurable. I responded with a resounding yes, of course, it's fantastic. She retorted with, "Well, you could have fooled me. You are just lying there like a corpse, not giving me any verbal indication that you are enjoying the experience." I was so into what she was doing that I was silently enjoying my experience. This didn't work for her because her dominant sense was auditory, and without auditory feedback from me, touching wasn't turning her on.

Once I realized that our dominant senses were different within the sexual context, I needed to translate my experience to the sense that was dominant for her. So, when she was touching me, I started to make verbal indications that what she was doing was pleasurable to me, and this auditory stimulation made her more excited. I didn't need to have a conversation, but I didn't lie there like a stiff, either. When you are interacting with a lover, ask them what they think their dominant sense is. That way, if you have a different dominant sense, you, too, will be able translate your sexual experience in a way that connects with them on a sensual level. It's just a lot more fun and fulfilling.

Works Cited

1. Kanner, Bernice. Are You Normal About Sex, Love, and Relationships? 2003, 52.
2. The Sexual Response Cycle. University of California–Santa Barbara, retrieved 2007-07-30.
3. Rathus, Spencer A., Nevid, Jeffrey S., Fichner-Rathus, Lois, Herold, Edward S., & McKenzie, Sue Wicks. Human Sexuality in a World of Diversity (2nd ed.). New Jersey: Pearson Education, 2005.
4. UCSB Sexinfo Online.
5. Slater, Philip E. "Sexual Adequacy in America." Intellectual Digest, Nov. 1973.
6. Sally Schloss for WebVet.
7. Pheromones in Humans: Myth or Reality? ©1992 David Wolfgang-Kimball.
8. Sources: UN Development Programme (UNDP). Human Development Report 1998. (New York: Oxford University Press, 1998), pp. 30 through 37. Published in World Watch Magazine, January/February 1999, Vol. 12, No. 1.
9. http://intimacy-sex.knoji.com/sex-and-the-five-senses/
10. UCSB Sexinfo Online.
11. http://sexualcommunication.wikispaces.com/Kaplan%E2%80%99s+Triphasic+Model
12. Zilbergeld, Bernie. The New Male Sexuality. New York: Bantam Books, 1992.
13. Sex and the Five Senses. James R. Coffey, Yahoo Contributor Network. Sep. 15, 2010. http://voices.yahoo.com/sex-five-senses-6796224.html

6

Whose Job is it Anyway?

Pleasure and Responsibility

Who is responsible for the quality and satisfaction of a couple's sexual experience? Who is responsible to initiate and orchestrate the event? Generally students and patients respond that both members are equally responsible for happens during the sexual experience. Ideally, that's the right answer, but in our culture, the male usually believes that he is responsible. Just by virtue of his sex, he is the one in charge of what is supposed to happen and be held accountable for the outcome of the experience. He is the sex expert because he is the man. He believes that it is his job to make his partner sexually happy by providing big orgasms—and lots of them.

I always joke that males are sex experts regarding female sexuality as well as their own because they "hung out" in the boys' locker room, learning about sex from their peers, and about women specifically. My generation read sex magazines like *Playboy* and *Penthouse* for their education. Today, many young males look to the Internet for all their great sex information, and they are able view so much explicit sexual activity of all kinds online—something that we could not even imagine before the Internet. Does all this access to sexual information make men more knowledgeable regarding sex? I don't think so. Most men don't know much about sex, and especially about female sexuality.

What is at stake psychologically for a male to take on a sense of sexual responsibility that he knows nothing about? In his mind, it's his sexual self-esteem, his masculinity, being an adequate lover and/or husband. Make no mistake: this responsibility isn't a superficial psychological issue.

When a man has the cognitive belief that he is responsible for his partner's sexual fulfillment and doesn't have the intimate sexual knowledge of his partner, this sets him up for a major psychological double bind. One key symptom of this bind is a great deal of anxiety. When anxiety and a sexual experience co-exist, the pleasure of the experience is removed. The double bind of sexual responsibility makes it very difficult for a man to relax during his lovemaking experience, which can affect his level of pleasure and ability to perform. It's as if he is on stage and is supposed to know his lines without anyone giving him the script.

Before the feminist movement of the 1970s, a popular belief was that men didn't care about their partner's sexual fulfillment. Enjoying sex was for the man, and children and family was for the woman. Men were just selfish about sex.

Women and Sexual Responsibility

Let's leave the man for a moment and look at how women relate to the issue of sexual responsibility. Many women in our culture relate to sexual responsibility in one of two ways. The first type is a woman who has little or no knowledge of her own sexuality. She feigns ignorance of what's below her waist and what her genitals are all about. She knows little about her own body and her own sexuality. But she doesn't have to despair. Coming to her rescue, in all his glory, is the male "expert" we have just discussed. He will teach her all about sex and her own body—or so she would like to believe.

This type of woman is perfect for our male sex expert because she is untainted, virginal, ready and willing to learn all that he can teach her—and without too much contradiction or conflict. Our expert feels safe and secure, because his sexual expertise is never questioned.

I don't see this type of woman in my clinical practice as often as I once did, which shows how women have changed sexually since the onset of the feminist movement. The myth of the male sexual expert has been exposed and has created psychological issues for many men who believe they still should be the experts.

A woman who is ignorant about her own sexuality is unable to take responsibility for her sexual needs and wants because she doesn't know herself. Unfortunately, she and her partner may become very frustrated and bored sexually, because their sexual relationship turns into the blind leading the blind.

There is a second kind of woman who is just the opposite of the one just discussed. She knows all about her body and her own sexuality. She learned how to experience sexual pleasure through masturbation or previous sexual experiences with other men, or both. She knows what her sexual needs and wants are. She knows what feels good, and she knows what would make her feel even better.

A woman who knows about her body sexually may find herself in a couple of psychological double binds. The first relates to her partner's fantasy that his partner is a virgin and hasn't been with other men before him. Even though he may know on a conscious level that she has been with other men sexually, he may still want to deny that this is true. If his partner starts taking responsibility for what happens sexually within their relationship, this may break his denial, forcing him to work through his emotional issue that she has had previous sexual experience.

Besides wrecking her partner's fantasy that she hasn't had any previous sexual experiences, the woman may be afraid to assert herself sexually and take responsibility for fear of being judged as a "bad girl" or worse, a slut. These fears may go back to early adolescence.

I remember back in high school that there were some girls, and even groups of girls, that everyone called whores or sluts. I never could understand why they were called this, because they didn't really seem to fit the image. They didn't walk around in fancy or sexy clothes or drive expensive cars, or charge for their sexual favors. Yet their peers put them down. Now, looking back, I realize that these girls may simply have been more sexually developed than the other, more immature girls and boys.

The conflict for some women is that if they don't take the psychological risk of asserting themselves sexually to improve their experience, they run the risk of upsetting their partner. The other choice is to inhibit themselves sexually so their partner can remain in denial about their sexual past. Enabling this denial will never work; taking the risk of asserting yourself has a much better chance of success.

The second double bind for a woman who takes responsibility for herself sexually is the concern of threatening her partner's sense of himself sexually. If a woman gives her partner any kind of suggestions or directions about what she would like sexually, she runs the risk that her partner will feel threatened and get angry and upset. He might react and say something like: "I don't need you to tell me how to make love to you. I am not inexperienced; I don't need a sex teacher in bed." His reaction stems from his belief that he is responsible for his partner sexually, and as a man, he knows what to do and shouldn't have to be told. Of course, the reality is that he doesn't know what to do, but he doesn't want to admit this. As they say, men don't like to ask for directions; they want to figure it out themselves, but all they do is end up going around in circles, lost and very frustrated. This same dynamic can happen sexually if they inhibit their partner from expressing herself sexually. If a sexually responsible woman doesn't express her unique sexual desires and needs, her motivation to participate in sexual activity within that relationship will likely be diminished. It is just not fulfilling or that much fun for her to go around in circles and end up getting sexually frustrated.

The belief that a man is responsible for what happens sexually is unproductive and destined to lead to trouble. What works, then? Simply this: the woman is responsible for herself—and her partner is responsible for himself. If you are a man reading this book, you are the foremost authority on your own sexuality and body. You know what feels pleasurable and what doesn't, and that's really as far as your innate knowledge about sex goes. I don't care how many women you have been with sexually. It doesn't matter how many books you have read or classes that you have taken. You still don't really have any inherent sexual knowledge about the woman that you are involved with. I am a sex therapist, and a professor of human sexuality. I have studied female sexual anatomy and physiology, and I still don't know about my wife's specific likes and dislikes in the moment unless she tells me what they are. Knowing your partner's needs and desires will make you an effective, sensitive, caring lover. And only she can provide you with that information.

The reason a man doesn't know about a woman's specific sexual needs is that every woman is different sexually, and every woman is different at any given time. The reality is that no set pattern or technique works to satisfy your partner. Some men say that when they discover some way of pleasing their partner, they keep trying to repeat that pattern, but they get frustrated because it doesn't produce the same result. Even when their partner tells them to do something different, they just go back to the same sexual pattern, frustrating their partner and eventually themselves. When a man believes that he is sexually responsible for his partner's sexual satisfaction, it's difficult psychologically to take risks and break away from a pattern that has been successful in the past with other women or his current lover.

The psychological upside of the fact that every woman is unique regarding her sexual desires and needs, and that the same woman can be sexually different from one experience to another, is that there is no predictability. Our hormones change. Our moods change. Our likes and dislikes change. We're fortunate that this is so; otherwise, our sex lives would become predictable and boring.

The reality is that I don't know what my wife may like at any given time when I approach her sexually. I know some basic things, but for the specifics, I need some communication from her, either verbal or nonverbal. I need an open mind so I can be sensitive to the nuances of the moment. I need the "map to the territory."

You don't follow the same path to sexual fulfillment every time you make love. This creates a certain amount of excitement and a sense of the unknown, which breaks the cycle of doing the same thing repeatedly that results in sexual boredom. In order to enjoy this unpredictability, a man needs to let go of the belief that he must know what he is doing sexually with his partner without having the map to the territory. Otherwise, he is going to be a nervous wreck, full of performance anxiety and unable to enjoy and experience the pleasure of the moment.

To counter the sense of anxiety, some men develop a template approach to sexual interaction. They find a pattern of sexual stimulation that may have been successful with one particular lover, and then they apply the same pattern to all the other lovers with whom they have sexual encounters. It's as if they believe they have the magic formula to sexual fulfillment for all women and thus don't have to worry about performance. This takes away any sexual anxiety they might experience.

This template can also occur in a long-term marital relationship. A husband finds a pattern of stimulation that was very successful in pleasing his wife and then he follows that same pattern every time they make love. She tells him to try something else, but he keeps going back to that pattern, thinking that he will get the same result as he once did.

A man who operates sexually from a template might say something like, "Sally, I don't know what the problem is. This approach worked for Mary Jane. Why don't you like what I'm doing?" This sort of language implies that there is something wrong with Sally because she doesn't respond to his technique. The problem is obvious. The man is failing to see that Sally is not Mary Jane.

He doesn't understand that all women respond differently to sexual stimulation and the same woman may respond differently at any given time. What felt good last time may be irritating today. The man in this example is failing to recognize that everyone man and woman is sexually unique.

On a psychological level, the idea that someone is responsible for another adult in any form is problematic. This also holds true in the case of being responsible for another person's sexual fulfillment. When an individual believes they are responsible for their partner's sexuality, this sets them up to be the "psychological parent" in the relationship, making their partner a child psychologically within the sexual context.

This is what's called the classic co-dependent relationship. Some people find it less threatening to view their lover as a child, especially if they are insecure about their own sexuality and need a sense of control, but for most people, this type of relationship reeks of deeper underlying psychological problems. We aren't talking about a relationship between two equal adults when responsibility is involved. They may be adults chronologically, but not in terms of emotional development.

One of the psychological payoffs of being responsible for another adult is the sense of control. The problem is that when controlling behavior is involved with intimacy, whether emotionally or sexually, it has a detrimental impact. If an adult perceives that they are being controlled, they are likely to develop a great deal of resentment, which will result with an inhibited sexual desire.

Another factor that occurs when controlling behavior becomes part of a sexually intimate relationship is a lack of psychological vulnerability. Adults generally don't want to open up and let go emotionally or physically when someone is trying to control them. Without vulnerability, the potential for sexual passion and excitement are going to fade between the couple over time.

Taking responsibility for your partner's sexual experience also sets you up for feeling emotionally angry, frustrated and eventually very inadequate. Co-dependents, sexually or otherwise, see themselves as coming to their partner's rescue. They think they are going to fix any sexual problems and give their partner some amazing sexual experience. This all sounds well intended, but the problem is that they don't have the power or ability to achieve any of these goals. You can't make someone have a fantastic orgasm, no matter how good your technique might be. Your partner has the ultimate control over how they are going to respond to sexual stimulation.

The anger and resentment that comes from the co-dependent's doomed efforts to make their partner happy sexually are usually directed at their partner. Getting mad at their partner just makes the atmosphere between them more anti-erotic, and makes the situation worse when it comes to the potential for sexual fulfillment.

A classic example is where a wife believes she can fix her husband's erection difficulty by doing things sexually that she thinks should turn him on. She might buy sexy lingerie at Victoria's Secret, thinking this might help the problem, but instead this backfires and her partner perceives her effort as more pressure, creating more performance anxiety for him. This in turn makes it more difficult for him to get an erection. His wife gets mad that she is making efforts to "fix" the problem and directs her anger at her husband, which again only compounds the erection difficulty. The woman in this case needs to learn that she can't fix her partner's sexual problem—only he can do that, with her help. Only he can prescribe the remedy to his problem.

When both partners believe that they are responsible for each other's sexual experience, they create the perfect setup for sexual frustration and disappointment. If we put a couple in bed together with all their programming about sexual responsibility the following scenario can occur.

The male partner is like an airplane pilot flying in the fog without any instruments. He touches his partner in one spot and then another, hoping that he is doing the right thing. But, of course, he keeps his feelings of uncertainty to himself. On the surface, everything is under control; he is the expert and he knows what he is doing. Below the surface, he is experiencing considerable anxiety and frustration because not only are his pride and ego at stake, but so is the continuation of his relationship with his lover. He is caught in a double bind. On one hand, he wants the sexual experience to be mutually satisfying; on the other, he can't really let himself go and express himself honestly and spontaneously, because he would then be admitting that he really doesn't know what he is doing. He is setting himself up for failure.

His sexual companion is probably saying to herself, "God, I wish he would get it together and do it right!" This is particularly true if this woman is ignorant of her own body, since she is depending on him to know what he is doing sexually. Now she is finding out that he is not the expert she thought or hoped he was. The woman who knows what she likes sexually may be equally frustrated because she feels inhibited in communicating what she wants for the reasons discussed earlier.

For both the man and woman in this scenario, their sexual experience is frustrating and anxiety producing. But given their programming, they are unable to communicate. So, they keep making love—with increased frustration and disappointment. Finally, they get to the point where it is less painful simply to avoid sex, so the frequency of their sexual activity decreases. Sometimes this couple might stumble upon a way of interacting sexually that works, but they tend to stick to the new method until they've worn it out, too. Then they find themselves frustrated and bored to the point where the frequency of their sexual activity decreases even more.

In his book, *Male Sexuality,* Bernie Zilbergeld puts it this way: "The man not only conducts the band, but he also plays all the instruments too." (1) The concept that the man is responsible for his own and his partner's sexuality is a barrier to creating a satisfying sexual experience for either of them. The only way that this concept could work is if somehow we could connect the nerve endings in the woman's genitals to the man's brain. Then if he needs to be responsible for her satisfaction, he could be aware of her experience, at least technically. However, there are better, more realistic ways to give each other sexual pleasure.

Now that we have discussed the concept of sexual responsibility, it becomes clear how absurd it is for one adult to be responsible for another's subjective experience, be it around sex or any other part of an adult relationship. But what does it mean to take responsibility for your own sexuality? This phrase can sound so much like "psychobabble." What does it really mean in everyday life? On a behavioral level, taking responsibility for your own sexuality means using the communicative phrase: "**I want....**" or "**I don't want....**" within a sexual context.

By using these communicative phrases, the speaker is communicating in an adult, assertive manner. Using "I" messages is a way to take care of yourself sexually. These statements are not demands; they are more like requests that are always negotiable. Demanding is unacceptable behavior between two equal adults.

Some perceive that "I" messages sound selfish. They are only selfish if the sender wants what they want regardless of how their partner feels emotionally about giving them what they want. "I want" statements are a gift to me because they give me a way to pleasure my partner, which in turn will give me a great deal of pleasure as well. It can be a win-win for both partners, as long as there is choice in doing what the other partner wants. If it's forced, pressured, demanded, or manipulated, then it's not a gift and the resentment from the attempt to control will build over time, which may lead to the dissolution of the relationship, at least as lovers.

Using "I" statements puts the sender in a psychologically vulnerable position. To take the risk and communicate within the sexual context requires a great deal of trust between the couple. With this form of communication a couple will be able to give each other the "heads-up" about what their partner can do to make their sexual experience extremely pleasurable, and what things they can avoid doing that would turn their sexual experience unsatisfying.

If you don't know what you want, you can't ask for it. This couldn't apply more to what happens in a sexual relationship. So if you don't know what you want sexually then you need to do your own research and then you will be able to be sexually assertive and hence responsible for your own pleasure.

Trust and Responsibility

Many areas of trust play a critical role within an intimate relationship, but one key area is in the sexual context. Can you trust your lover or spouse to take responsibility for his or her sexuality? If you can, then you don't have to worry about guessing what he or she wants and needs. You have the basis for a high level of sexual pleasure within your relationship.

What I generally recommend to couples in order to establish this level of trust is to have a verbal **agreement** that they will each take care of themselves sexually by expressing what they both want or need in the moment—that they will communicate this information and therefore take responsibility for their own sexuality.

When this type of an agreement is not in place, you can't trust your partner to take responsibility for himself or herself. You will tend to become preoccupied with thinking about your partner's sexual experience. This kind of thinking is anything but an aphrodisiac. It usually runs along these lines: "I hope she likes what I'm doing to her," or "I'm afraid that I'm taking too long and that he's getting bored," or "I think she is just making love to me because she feels guilty." Such thoughts simply get in the way of feeling the pleasure of the moment, because they create so much performance anxiety.

A verbal agreement takes away the worries and associated anxiety about whether you are doing something right or wrong, because if your partner doesn't enjoy something you are doing, they will tell you, and if they want you to something that will make it better for them, they will give you that information as well. If they are not communicating any information, you can assume that whatever was occurring was just fine for them. If I can assume my wife is taking care of herself in this way, I don't have to think about her from a performance point of view. Instead, I am able to enjoy my own experience to its fullest. Knowing that, my wife becomes even more aroused so a very pleasurable synergetic effect is created.

One patient told me that when his wife was performing oral sex on him he believed that she was doing so only for his pleasure, and that she did not enjoy the experience. So, whenever he found himself in that sexual situation, he would start thinking about her not enjoying herself and would feel guilty. This quickly robbed him of the pleasure he might have experienced.

In a therapy session one day, he asked his wife, "Do you enjoy giving me pleasure that way?" And she replied "Sure, it turns me on to feel you getting so excited by something I'm doing. Plus I love you and I like to give you pleasure." Once he heard that, he stopped worrying about his partner and just enjoyed the experience to the fullest, confident that they were sharing a mutual pleasure.

What Type of Sexual Party Do You Want to Experience with Your Partner?

As a conclusion to the concept of sexual responsibility, I want to give a metaphorical example of a party as an illustration of what can happen sexually between a couple.

When you host a party for your friends, there are two kinds of parties you can give. In the first scenario, you prepare for the party days ahead of time and purchase the necessary items such as food and drinks. The day of the party you are setting up and preparing for your guests' arrival. When your friends finally arrive, you are constantly checking on them to make sure they have enough food and drink. You are introducing people to each other so they feel comfortable and involved in the party. You might try to get people to dance if that is one of the activities. As the host, you want everyone to have a good time and enjoy themselves.

If this seems like a lot of work, you might think twice about having another party in the near future. If you can afford it, you might consider hiring a party planner and a caterer so you won't have to do all the work. But you may still feel that you are responsible for everyone's good time.

Another way to give a party is to ask all of your guests to bring food and drinks, like a potluck. When your guests arrive, you greet them at the front door, telling them that food and drinks are in the kitchen. You tell them that there are all kinds of people to meet and just to say hello, that everyone is friendly. If they need anything else, you will be hanging out around the front door, so they can go and have a good time.

When the party is over, you aren't as exhausted because you didn't spend the whole time taking responsibility for everyone's good time. Unlike the first type of party style, you might want to give this party again. It was fun for the host as well as the guests.

When lovers take responsibility for their partners' sexual experience, they are like the first party host mentioned. Their sexual experience becomes a job—something they aren't going to be excited about being involved in, especially after working all day and when they are tired. You can choose what party host you would like to be.

Work Cited

1. Kanner, Bernice. Are You Normal About Sex, Love, and Relationships? 2003, 52.

7

The Concept of Sexual Goal Orientation

The cognitive concept of goal-oriented sex was something I learned indirectly from Masters and Johnson when I trained as a sex therapist. This concept has had major positive implications, both in my professional and personal lives. I hope that sharing this information will be as helpful for you in enhancing the level of pleasure in your personal life.

We are all familiar with goals—academic goals, professional goals, financial goals, and personal goals. In these areas of our lives, goals and goal setting can certainly be helpful. But when goals infiltrate our sexual lives, they create more problems than they solve. I've known couples who had small sexual goals that only mildly inhibited their sexual pleasure. And I've known couples who had large sexual goals that turned their sexual experience into a frustrating, disappointing, unfulfilling disaster. In my experience, when it comes to sex, more and bigger goals mean more and bigger problems.

What time frame do goals occupy—past, present, or future? Goals always relate to the future. If we are mentally in the future, then that means we're not in the present. In order to experience sexual pleasure to its fullest, it's essential to be mentally engaged in the present. When our attention drifts into the future, we become distracted. We start thinking about what's going to happen down the road. Some people—especially those who are very goal or success oriented in their lives in general—tend to worry so much about the future that they never get there. They miss all the pleasures of the moment. The future only exists in imagination. Seize the moment—that's where the fun is in life.

There is a local mountain near where I live called Mount Diablo. It's a California State Park. Many locals like to go up to the top and see the view from there, from which on a clear day, you can see for miles. Let's say we decided to hike up Mount Diablo one sunny day. But as we go along the trail up the mountain, we don't look at the flowers and the views along the way. We just keep wondering when we we'll get to the top and what we'll do when we get there. It seems as if the hike is taking a long time, and we aren't having that much fun or pleasure.

Finally, after hours of hiking, we get to the summit of Mount Diablo. Our goal of getting to the top has been achieved. We look at the view and visit the snack bar to get something eat and drink, and then it's time to go back down. We are now in a hurry to get down because we are tired, so again, we don't spend any time enjoying the hike down. It's all about the goal of getting down.

This story is a good illustration about how many people approach their lives. Did you achieve the goal, whatever that might be at the time? Once I was in a gift shop, and I saw a poster on the wall that said, "Life is a journey, not a destination." As John Lennon sang in "Beautiful Boy (Darling Boy" (1980), "Life is what happens to you while you're busy making other plans."

Both these quotes I think are important in the way we look at how we live our lives, but they are especially relevant to the approach we take to our sexual experience. It's all about the here and now, a phrase from the 1960s author, Ram Dass.(1) How relevant and needed this concept is in today's world that is telling us to hurry up and get it done already.

The antidote cognitive concept to goal orientation is that sex is about **the journey, not the destination**. The majority of the pleasure really lies in the process of getting to the goal, whatever that might be.

Is Foreplay Sex?

One word in our sexual vocabulary epitomizes this goal-oriented thinking: "foreplay." Foreplay, of course, is sexual activity such as kissing, hugging, fondling, holding, touching, and caressing; it also includes verbal expressions of endearment like, "I love you. You look really beautiful and sexy tonight." The words can refer to all kinds of tactile and verbal sensual stimulation of your lover.

When I ask patients or students what the purpose of foreplay is, they usually respond that it is something you do to get ready to have sex. What they are really saying is that foreplay is the preliminary to intercourse. The word itself implies this: foreplay by definition is play that goes before something else, and for most people, that something else is sex.

For teenagers or young adults who have not yet had their first experience of intercourse, foreplay is the sum total of the sexual activity that takes place. When I was a teenager, this was called making out; previous generations called it necking or petting. Whatever it was called, it was a great experience! We generally understood that intercourse wasn't yet acceptable.

When I had a girlfriend back then, I couldn't wait for Saturday night because that's when we would be together and hopefully make out in some private setting. All week leading up to Saturday night, I was trying to find a place where we could be alone in a private place that was comfortable for us to be together. There was no spontaneity operating in this case, although I might have acted as if I had no plans.

When the moment finally arrived, we would spend what seemed like hours touching each other, kissing each other in various states of undress, and getting very excited and aroused. Talk about a sensuous, pleasurable, erotic loving experience. We were totally in the present. We knew that we had arrived, and this was all that was going to happen. It was so pleasurable that I couldn't wait until the following Saturday night when we were going to have this experience all over again. Yes, you might say that this experience was frustrating because I might go home with wet underwear, but given the amount of pleasure that occurred, it was well worth it.

Something changes in a relationship once the "green light" is on, that it's okay to engage in intercourse. Once the couple is committed to each other or married and intercourse is possible, then all the foreplay they once enjoyed seems like some adolescent activity that is merely in the way of real adult sex—namely, intercourse.

I believe that the amount of time a couple spends involved with foreplay shrinks in direct proportion to the length of time they have been together. When the amount of foreplay decreases, the amount of time spent kissing, fondling, touching, and holding each other decreases. When this occurs, what's going out of the couple's sexual relationship? The answer is sensuality, touching, and real intimacy within the sexual context. They are no longer really making love—now they are just having sex.

When the amount of time a couple is involved in foreplay decreases, then the couple complains that marital sex is a bore and there isn't any "spice," just the same old thing. Well, the first remedy they might consider to this condition is to increase the quantity and quality of their touching and the amount of time they spend at foreplay, even to the point of agreeing that their involvement might not lead to intercourse. Just like when I used to make out on those Saturday night dates I mentioned earlier.

When foreplay becomes subordinate to the "big event"—intercourse—the sexual attitude of the couple begins to change. They start asking questions that are indicative of this attitude change such as: "Are you turned on yet?" "Are you ready?" "Come on, let's get it on," "I have to go to work tomorrow," "Good, let's stop this fooling around and have sex." The attitude is all about moving on to something in the future, and not just hanging out and enjoying the moment.

The big question that I like to ask groups when I am giving a seminar or when I am teaching a class is, "IS FOREPLAY SEX?" Most people will say no, it's not sex. Foreplay is something you do to have sex.

The answer is, of course, that foreplay *is* sex. It is a very sexual experience. If, during foreplay, you're thinking about the next step—intercourse—you have effectively removed yourself from the pleasure of the moment. While intercourse is an important part of sex, it is no more the whole of sex than the seeds are the whole of the apple.

So why do so many people believe that foreplay is not sex? The reason is that foreplay as a stand-alone experience isn't about sexual reproduction. Foreplay by itself is just about sexual pleasure and arousal. It doesn't produce babies. This is why when people say they had sex, it's always about the act of sexual intercourse. Our own President Clinton denied he had sex in the Oval Office because he was just involved with oral stimulation, and thus didn't have sex because he didn't participate in sexual intercourse.

Americans have a reproductive view of sex. Our culture has decided that only intercourse itself is "real sex." This idea may stem from past and current religious programming, which decreed that the only valid purpose for sex was reproduction. If sex is indeed for making babies, then intercourse is clearly the focus of sex. But if sex is for pleasure, then this type of thinking is obsolete.

Defining foreplay as something apart from, preliminary to, and less than full sex may be one of the single most destructive ideas our society has about sexual relations. This concept robs us of experiencing sexual pleasure to its fullest potential.

The Meat-and-Potatoes Sex Equation

Now that we have explored the first step—foreplay—let's follow the path to the next step in the pattern of typical goal-oriented sexual activity. The next stop on the journey is intercourse. When couples engage in sexual intercourse, do they focus on the pleasure of the moment? Do they see how long they can sustain pleasure while they are experiencing sexual intercourse? Generally, from my professional experience, it's about getting to the next goal—orgasm. It's so ironic that they make a big deal about getting to have intercourse when they are involved in foreplay, but when they finally get to intercourse, they seem to immediately focus on the next goal, orgasm.

They're thinking about "the Big O." They may be saying to themselves or to each other, "Did you come?" or "Uh-oh, I'd better slow down or I'm going to come," "I'm coming too fast," or "I'd better hurry up and come." This sort of dialogue focuses on the future, not the present, and reveals how the sexual pleasure of the moment is being missed. All they want to do is produce an orgasm.

Now, there is nothing wrong with wanting to experience an orgasm, but they generally are short lived. On average, a woman's orgasm lasts about 18 seconds and a man's last about 22 seconds. So we aren't talking about a whole lot of time of awesome sexual pleasure. It's over before you know it. Of course, women can experience one orgasm right after another, whereas males are limited to one.

Once a couple experiences orgasm, the sexual journey is over. They have reached the end of the line; they have achieved their goal. The question remains, what was their goal? Just to say they had sex, perhaps, but how much fun and pleasure was involved? It's not uncommon for someone to say to me, "What's the big deal about sex?" I can understand their question when you understand the way they psychologically approach the way they experience sex.

The reason for the couple's lack of pleasure during their sexual experience is due to the fact that whatever they were doing sexually was done to get to the next step along the way. Mentally, they were thinking about the goal of getting to the end, as opposed to enjoying the moment for its own sake.

The pattern I describe looks like this:

Foreplay + Intercourse = Orgasm

This pattern is the way that I think too many couples make love. I call this pattern meat-and-potatoes sex. There is nothing inherently wrong with this pattern, but after a couple of experiences of this type of goal-oriented sex, they might begin to wonder if they're missing something.

It's like eating fast food for the quick relief of one's hunger—it satisfies the appetite, but it doesn't provide much in the way of real nourishment. To draw a parallel, if a couple's sex life is made up of fast food, they may suffer from a different kind of malnourishment, called pleasure deprivation. While there is nothing wrong with a "quickie" now and then, when goal-oriented sex becomes more the rule than the exception, it's time to take a new look at what you're doing sexually.

The Attitudes of Goal-Oriented Sex

One common belief is that once a couple engages in foreplay or touching each other, it must lead to intercourse, which, in turn, ends with an orgasm. It's as if the couple gets on a train in San Francisco going all the way to New York, without any stopovers or side trips. That would be fine if it happens to be a business trip. But if the whole purpose of the trip is pleasure, wouldn't it make more sense to let the journey unfold at its own pace and in its own way? Maybe the highlight of the entire trip is a canyon in Utah or a waterfall in Colorado. Maybe we don't need to "go all the way" to New York at all!

In *Male Sexuality*, Bernie Zilbergeld says that a common male sexual myth is that good sex is a linear progression of increasing excitement, terminating in orgasm. Sex, according to this view, should be a process of continually increasing excitement and passion. Sexual arousal should continue to build. Not only must we go all the way, but we must do so with a certain speed and intensity, somewhat like a steam train leaving the station. But when we pursue sex with this kind of goal orientation, our sexual relationship becomes rigid; and when rigidity sets in, the relationship becomes predictable and boring. Foreplay, intercourse, and orgasm over and over again. It's like following the same path in the Sierra Nevada mountains. When you're on the path, you feel a certain amount of security and safety. If you lose the path, you're flooded with anxiety, but at the same time, it's exciting exploring new territory with new discoveries. For some couples, it's just safer to stay rigid than to move into new sexual territory.

When I work with couples trying to improve their sex lives, I try to therapeutically break up their rigid pattern and help them develop greater flexible ways of interacting sexually. Remember, rigidity equals boredom, so my therapeutic goal is to take away their predictability. When I suggest to couples that they learn to be more flexible in their sex life, they immediately picture weird and kinky activities. I'm not adverse to such activities if the couple can be comfortable with them, but you don't have to go to extremes just to break the monotony!

I often advise people who are caught in the meat-and-potatoes routine to vary the sexual options they currently enjoy. I suggest that they treat sex as a leisurely activity, with breaks for resting, laughing, and talking. And I introduce the possibility that orgasm doesn't have to be the main goal. Many couples learn that their greatest sexual pleasure comes when they concentrate most of their attention on kissing, fondling, and touching each other. Maybe this activity flows into intercourse, and then goes back to kissing and touching again. They might also touch and kiss each other to the point of mutual satisfaction, having orgasms manually or orally, never engaging in intercourse.

In other words, breaking up the foreplay-plus-intercourse-equals-orgasm equation and the habit of goal-oriented sex opens doors to whole vistas of possibility. A couple may start to feel that they don't do the same thing twice. When improvisation is a part of the sexual experience, it allows for creativity and the excitement of the unknown potential, no matter how long a couple has been making love to one another.

Sex Doesn't End with Orgasm

Another example of rigidity in a relationship—and one that puts a great deal of emotional pressure on men—is when the man ejaculates before his partner has experienced an orgasm. Often, once the male ejaculates, the whole sexual experience comes to a crashing halt. The man says, "I'm tired now, I'm going to sleep," or, "I'm sorry, maybe next time." Why is this? If it is 1:00 P.M., why is he going to sleep? I know that a male ejaculation can be intense, but so much so that he has to go to sleep in the middle of the day? I think something else is going on here.

The answer is psychological. I could understand being sleepy if it was 1:00 A.M. after a long day of activity, but that's not the case here. Because of this tendency, women sometimes think of men as sexually selfish because they don't seem to care about their partner's satisfaction. Whether he is, in fact, being selfish or not (and this is, no doubt, sometimes the case), the man may also retire from sex play out of a feeling of inadequacy.

Many men, and women, too, have a rigid idea of how they are supposed to experience orgasm. The man may think that once he ejaculates and loses his erection, he will be unable to pleasure and satisfy his partner, because he believes that the only right or normal way to stimulate a woman to orgasm is with his penis. Once he has ejaculated, if he is unable to have another erection right away, he feels inadequate and embarrassed. He wants to escape the situation, which may be why he wants to go to sleep.

Rigid thinking of this kind limits our sexual experiences and puts unnecessary pressure on us, which, of course, only further limits the amount of sexual pleasure we can experience. Philip Slater said it best in his article, "Sexual Adequacy in America": "The antidote to this type of thinking would be to view orgasm as a delightful interruption in an otherwise continuous process of generating pleasurable sensations. This would break the habit of looking at orgasm as a unit to be quantified as in 'we made love three times, he has two cars.'"(2)

A more flexible attitude, and one that allows for more pleasure, might be the following: whatever way a woman can experience orgasm is right and normal. So, if a man loses his erection after ejaculation, what's wrong with using his hands or mouth to stimulate his partner? Either of these methods might be as pleasurable for her as intercourse. Once again, this need not evolve into another rigid pattern, but it certainly gives the man more options and the relationship more variety.

A woman in this situation can ask her partner to give her more stimulation so that she won't feel frustrated and possibly resentful. She may even do so by initiating further touching or performing oral sex on him if he is open to further penis stimulation. If this is done in a loving and sensitive way, making sure the man understands that she still perceives him to be sexy and a source of erotic stimulation, she may avoid the problems that flow from the man feeling inadequate.

Sexual Goals and Performance Anxiety

In addition to distracting us from the present, sexual goals create another major problem—emotional anxiety. When people really want to succeed at achieving a goal like passing a final exam, they experience a great deal of anxiety or nervousness before the experience and while it occurs. When you really want to do well, or you know your score on a test will make the difference between a final grade of A or B, how do you feel emotionally? You probably feel nervous, pressured, and anxious. The anxiety can be so severe that it can cripple the individual from performing the task at hand. These same emotions and conditions can inhibit sexual pleasure.

Usually, when a couple "work" at trying to improve their sexual relationship, the harder they try, the worse the problem becomes. Finally, they may simply give up working at their sex life out of pure frustration and disappointment.

Typically, we are told that if we have a problem, all we need to do is try harder and apply ourselves, and we will overcome and succeed at resolving the problem. With many things in life, this attitude may be true. This really is the case with successful people who have achieved their goals in life. They succeeded at achieving the goals through hard work and perseverance. This approach to life paid off for them in a major way, but it is these high achievers who are highly susceptible to sexual difficulties.

The reason for this is that what worked for them in life in general doesn't work at all in their sexual life. It is the total opposite. The goal-oriented person can be so caught up in attaining future rewards—and in delaying their immediate gratification in favor of a bigger prize—that they forget that sex is about pleasure and enjoyment in the here and now.

The harder an individual or couple **works** at making their sexual relationship better, the worse it gets. This belief is completely different from how most of us were taught. In order to improve your sex life, you want to get the concept of work out of the experience. When you listen to the language people use when referring to their sexual life, you can hear the work ethic. They use such goal-oriented phrases as, "We need to *make* love," "I need to *perform* sexually tonight," "I have to *produce* an erection," "I need to *achieve* an orgasm, or he will be upset." I get exhausted just listening to these phrases. The problem is that couples are turning something that's supposed to be fun, pleasurable, and relaxing into a work experience.

Work and sexual pleasure are natural enemies, and the more personal the commitment to work, the more inroads it makes into one's sexual life. If people work all day at their jobs or raising children (or both), by the time their day comes to an end, I don't think they will be excited about going to bed with the expectation that they have to work some more in terms of their sexual life.

As a consequence of these work/goal-oriented sexual attitudes, couples' sexual frequency decreases. One classic example of this situation is when a couple is trying to have a baby and they work really hard at getting pregnant. They make sure it is the right time of the month, the right hour of the day, and they check her temperature to see if she is ovulating. When all those variables are in correct alignment, then it's time to have intercourse—whether they really feel like it or not. Again, something that is supposed to be fun and relaxing becomes work—a goal-oriented experience. If you are one of the many people who have done this, it may take you a while to enjoy sex again after the goal of reproduction has been achieved.

Often, in my clinical practice, I see women with small children; they have very little or no interest in being sexually involved with their husbands. If I write on a piece of paper: sex = __________ and ask them what they would put in the blank, they usually say work or another job. Taking care of small children all day can be incredibly draining. By the time a young mother who stays at home with her small children has all her tasks done for the day and has her kids asleep for the night, the last thing on her mind is sex.

When the woman gets into bed, the first thing on her husband's mind is sex, and he starts to initiate. She usually responds with "I am tired," and the conflict of desire ensues. She views sex at this point as another situation where she has to put out more energy and give to her husband. But she has been putting out energy all day, and in the evening when she gets to bed, this is the last thing she wants to do. By saying no to her husband, she is also saying no to herself. She is cutting off one of the few—and probably the best—opportunities to experience pleasure.

One way that I try to help change this situation is first to have the mother in this case change her belief that she has to put out more energy, but instead view being sexual with her husband as an opportunity to receive energy—a time for her to be given to and recharge her batteries. I'm sure her husband would like to give to her in a physical and pleasing way, compared to the alternative of having no sexual interaction. Of course, this would require that she could keep her eyes open and be conscious.

Goal-oriented sexuality can greatly interfere with the frequency of sex, even with couples without children or whose children are grown. Often, a lover will say, "I am too tired tonight, honey," but then stay up and look at their tablet or watch television instead. This sort of response and action makes sense to the person who views a sexual relationship as a series of goals to be achieved. After working all day trying to produce, perform, and achieve, the last thing such a person would want to do is to continue working when they were finally at home and going to bed.

Sex, Relaxation, and Pleasure

Some of my better times sexually have been when I'm physically tired, such as after skiing all day, or playing tennis, or jogging. After I have skied all day or played tennis and I am at home, I take a nice long shower or sit in my spa. After that, usually I have a nice dinner, and after dinner I am relaxed physically, but mentally alert. Being relaxed is the key to sexual pleasure. We are at our best when there is no pressure to put on a sexual production or performance, when we are simply being open to receiving and giving sexual pleasure. I view sexual pleasure as a way of reenergizing myself. Instead of being an energy-draining experience, it's a way to recharge myself. Christiane Northrup, MD, author of *Women's Bodies, Women's Wisdom*, states that, "sexual energy is one of our most powerful energies for creating health. By using sexual energy consciously ... we can tap into a true source of youth and vitality."(3)

Incredible though it may seem, many people have difficulty accepting the idea that we should allow ourselves to have pleasure. I ask couples: "How much pleasure do you have in your life?" I don't mean the kind of pleasure that you experience by working at something like gardening or running five miles—this is (to varying degrees) a goal-oriented activity. I mean the kind of pleasure in which you are able to just kick back and enjoy an experience without having to produce or achieve anything—the kind of pleasure you get from just sitting on a beach or relaxing in a hot tub.

One Key to Great Sex: Flexibility

A flexible attitude toward the ways in which they make love to each other is extremely beneficial for a couple. Suppose that Jane is physically tired from the day's activities, but John has more energy; he does the initiating and more of the giving sexually, while Jane allows herself mostly to receive pleasure. On another occasion, the situation could be just the reverse. Sometimes, they may both have a lot of energy and will both be very involved in giving and receiving; sometimes, both are tired and just hold and touch each other because neither has much energy to give.

Again, the key to a vibrant sex life is flexibility. Sexual goals create a sense of rigidity, which limits your sexual expression and behavior. Rigidity cripples you sexually, preventing you from varying your sexual behavior to adapt to the varying conditions that occur over the course of a long-term relationship.

Flexibility in the way a couple interacts sexually also allows for the development of something called synergy. Synergy is a word coined by Carl Jung, the noted psychological theorist. He describes a synergistic situation, in which two systems working together produce results greater than the sum of their actions when working separately. Synergy occurs frequently in a relationship that is healthy and vibrant, and the word is especially apt in describing a fulfilling and pleasurable sexual exchange. Because synergy is, by definition, more than the logical combination of the parts, it is not something that can be decreed or prescribed. It comes upon you unexpectedly, and is thus synonymous with flexibility and openness.

An Awareness Experience: Moving from Goals to the Pleasure of the Moment

It is easy to see how goal orientation stands in the way of sexual pleasure in the moment. But we are a very goal-oriented society, and this way of thinking is deeply ingrained in us. How can we free ourselves of it? One way is by getting in touch with the primal sensations of our bodies.

In recent years, psychotherapists have learned that there are simple mental techniques that can be used to renew our focus on bodily sensations that might otherwise be blocked by our thoughts. The following is an exercise I've found to be most helpful for couples and individuals with whom I have worked clinically. I also use it myself when I need to focus my attention on the present.

To prepare yourself, get into a comfortable position, either sitting in a chair with both feet on the floor and hands resting gently on your knees, or lying on your back, hands at your sides and legs uncrossed. If you can do so, have a friend or your lover read the following instructions all the way through so you can become completely familiar with them before you start. You may then wish to keep this book beside you, with this exercise marked so that you can easily refer to it as you go along.

Take your time. Do each part of this exercise in a slow and leisurely way. Close your eyes, and let them stay closed until you finish this exercise. Stay at each step until you feel ready to move to the next. There is no time frame, only what seems right to you.

Okay, are you ready to begin? First, turn your attention to the way your body feels. Say out loud the different things you feel inside your body. Be as specific as you can. If you are doing the exercise by yourself, say your awareness to yourself. For example, you might say, "I feel tension in my neck," or "I feel the weight of my wristwatch on my arm." Say whatever you feel, describing whatever sensations you experience, no matter how insignificant they may seem to you.

As you become conscious of the different feelings in your body, let yourself be aware of your environment. Describe your awareness of what your senses are receiving in that environment. For example, you might say, "I'm aware of my neighbor mowing his lawn," or, "I'm aware of the children playing in the next room." Take your time and explore your awareness of the environment, verbally describing your awareness.

Now, express aloud all the thoughts that you are thinking. Say out loud everything that crosses your mind such as, "I'm thinking about eating dinner," or even "I'm thinking about thinking." Take your time. Explore and verbalize your thoughts in a leisurely way. Notice if you become conscious of any thoughts that you censor or repress back into your unconscious.

Turn your attention once more to what you feel in your body. Notice any changes from the first time you focused on your body. Have parts relaxed that were tense before? See if you can become aware of even the smallest of sensations, such as the pressure of your glasses on your nose, the slight tingling of your necklace around your neck, or the rhythmic expansion and contraction of your breathing.

Now, when you are ready, you can open your eyes.

Generally, when people have finished this awareness experience, they feel much more relaxed than when they started because they have acknowledged the messages that their bodies are sending them.

One major point of this exercise is to allow you to explore the three things on which you can focus your attention during your daily activities:

1. Your body's feelings or sensations;
2. Your awareness of the environment around you; and
3. Your thoughts.

Sensation, awareness, and thinking constitute three levels of consciousness. We go in and out of these different modes of awareness constantly, and the amount of time we spend in one or another can vary tremendously. When I am driving on the freeway, hopefully, my awareness is focused on what is going on around me, but I am sure you might have had the experience when you were deep in thought and drove past your exit. This is why texting while driving is so dangerous.

Contrary to the common assumption, we have a choice about which conscious mode we are in at any given moment. It's called selective attention. One application of this exercise is when you might be having trouble sleeping, and you wish you could just turn your brain off so you can fall asleep. This happens to me after I have given a seminar in the evening and it's 11:00 P.M., and I need to go to sleep because I have patient at 9:00 A.M. My mind is going over the whole seminar experience while I am lying down wanting to go to sleep. I use the exercise I just described and I focus on my body—and before I know it, I am asleep. I shift my mental focus on to my body's sensations and stop the thoughts that are keeping me awake.

Choosing Your Focus of Consciousness

During sexual activity, if you are touching or being touched and you are in thinking mode, it will be difficult for you to really feel the touch. This is what happens when sexual goals get involved because goals are all about thinking and not feeling the moment. In addition, if, while touching or being touched, you are aware of what your partner is doing, as if you were a spectator, or if you focus your attention on sounds coming from another room, it will likewise be difficult for you to enjoy the touching you are giving or receiving from your partner. If you are in the body sensations mode, then you will feel the stimulation to its fullest.

If a male's goal is not to have an orgasm before his partner, the whole time he's making love to his partner, he will be thinking about his goal. Just telling him to relax and not think about his goal won't work. He needs to mentally focus on something else, in this case what he is feeling with his body in the moment.

The most pleasurable mode of consciousness for sex is the feeling or body sensations mode. You want to be aware of all the sensations you feel—warmth, coolness, the smooth or rough parts of the body, the texture of hair, and so on. Too often, couples overlook these sensations and only seek orgasm—"the big turn-on." They are so caught up in achieving the goal that they miss all the pleasure along the way. What we are talking about here is sensuality, a key ingredient that is missing in the sexual relationships of all too many couples.

During sex, you may be focusing on your body feelings, but thoughts or awareness of the environment may distract you. If this occurs, simply acknowledge the thought or awareness. As strange as this may sound, that is the best way to free yourself from the interference. Let yourself become aware of the intruding thought or awareness, and then let it go, by focusing on what your body is feeling sexually. The choice is yours, not your body's.

When people are sexually goal oriented, where is their mental focus? They are into thinking. They are thinking about achieving the goal. All this thinking gets in the way of experiencing the feelings of pleasure in the moment. As a consequence, they most likely won't get to their sexual goal. This goal orientation is a basic component of most sexual problems.

After they've been together a few years, some couples tend to forget how they once were able to be sexually involved in many unlikely places, with many distractions in the environment—when they were parking by the side of the road; in the college dorm room; in her parents' living room when the rest of the family was (hopefully) asleep; and so on. It didn't seem to matter then that the conditions weren't ideal. Why? Because the desire to share physical intimacy with the other person was far stronger than any inhibiting distraction from the environment.

Interest overcomes obstacles. When we're listening to a speaker who is boring and speaks in a monotone, we may fidget and daydream; the least disturbance seizes our attention. But a dynamic speaker keeps us on the edge of our seat, and at the end of the talk, we don't know where the time went. The same principle applies to a sexual relationship. When someone has to have all the conditions absolutely perfect in order to be engaged sexually, it can be fruitful to ask if that person truly wants to be sexually involved in the first place.

Some people find that small amounts of alcohol or marijuana help them focus on the feelings they are experiencing during sex. They describe themselves as being "loose" after indulging—more able to be involved in the pleasure of the moment.

Drugs can shut off the "critical parent" in your thinking—the part of you that is full of don'ts and shoulds. It allows the natural child in you to be more spontaneous and uninhibited, to just let go and flow with what feels pleasurable, without passing judgment on whether it's right or wrong, good or bad. Drugs can act as a shortcut in developing this type of sexual freedom. I don't advocate the use of drugs or alcohol for better sex, because then an individual becomes dependent on a substance to have better sex. I would want to be able to achieve a sense of psychological/sexual freedom without the use of drugs. This state of being can be achieved through the awareness of the factors outlined in the experience above.

Our bodies are wonderful teachers, and our brains naturally contain all the chemical ingredients necessary to a blissful experience. As you free yourself from the sexual problems that your upbringing or society may have implanted, you are free to experience the full extent of sexual pleasure, without any artificial stimulation. With this knowledge, you possess a biological pharmacology of pleasure that no amount of artificial chemical stimulation through drugs or alcohol can give you, and it's all built right into your system. The good news is that there are no side effects or hangovers when you use your body to experience pleasure.

Works Cited

4. Dass, Ram. *Be Here Now.* New York: Crown Publishing Group, 1971.
5. Slater, Philip. "Sexual Adequacy in America." *Intellectual Digest,* Nov. 1973, pp. 17–22.
6. Northrup, Christiane, MD. *Women's Bodies, Women's Wisdom, Creating Physical and Emotional Health and Healing.* New York: Bantam Books, 2010.

8

Initiating Sexual Interaction

Many people, single and married alike, find it difficult to initiate sex. Sexual initiation is often the key to a couple's entire sexual relationship, since it is the moment when the decision is made to create that relationship. When the frequency of sex diminishes, initiation is one of the first things I explore with the couple in therapy. But initiation may be an issue, even if sex is not infrequent.

In our culture, we have many dos and don'ts about initiation, rules that structure and limit it. Who wrote these rules? It doesn't really matter where the rules came from—we needn't blindly adhere to them. If the rules get in our way, we are free as adults to rewrite them.

In Chapter One on sexual history, we looked at how our early concepts about sex are implanted. One of the first concepts that boys and girls often learn about sex is that men should be aggressive and women should be passive. I first learned this in a fifth grade dance class, where it was made quite clear that I was expected to ask the girl to dance, not the other way around.

I can still remember the anxiety I felt. Little did I know that this was the beginning of my education in sexual relations with women. And I can only imagine how uncomfortable it was for many of the girls to sit and wait, hoping that someone would ask them to dance. If they were not asked, they must have felt inadequate and publicly humiliated. There was the girl that none of us boys wanted to dance with—she was seen as "creepy." I feel sorry for her now and how she must have felt. From my perspective, all the girls looked cool as ice. I was the one who was insecure and nervous—or so I thought.

And so, a precedent was set. The seeds of some basic beliefs were planted—that the man—if he really is a man—is always trying to "get" the girl; meanwhile, she is always saying no to his advances, trying to act passive, disinterested, and cool. This is the classic sexual "dance" that men and women have played out through the ages. According to this scenario, men are programmed to initiate. A man is supposed to come on to the woman and make things happen—ask her out for a date, and then push her to have sex with him. A woman, on the other hand, can't act too interested; otherwise, she won't be seen as a "nice girl." Instead, she might be judged as a slut or a whore.

Many women are concerned about how they come across to men. They don't want to appear pushy or come on too strong for fear of being labeled aggressive. Les Parrot, professor of psychology at Seattle Pacific University and author of a new book called *Crazy Good Sex*, says that failing to initiate sex is one of the biggest mistakes women make.

"Most guys feel like they are always the initiator and that sets up disequilibrium on the passion scale in the relationship,"(1) he says. Generally, men want to be pursued by their partners just as much as women do.

I think the old stereotype that women are passive sexually has changed a great deal in the last 20 years. It seems that younger women are more comfortable with their sexuality and are more willing to go after what they want.

When there is a reversal of the old stereotype and the woman is sexually assertive while the man is passive, other people tend to judge them in various ways. All sorts of threats and fears come into play. "You don't want to threaten the man again and have him lose his erection now, do you?" "Do you want to be seen as a slut?" "You don't want him to think you push this hard with all the men you meet."

Society Discourages Assertive Women

It's just not generally acceptable for a woman to be sexually assertive in our society. While some women have succeeded in liberating themselves from this sexist stereotyping, it is very much alive in Western culture as a whole.

I am reminded again of the girls in my high school who were labeled whores. Other girls and boys who would put these particular girls down because they wore too much makeup or provocative clothing and teased their hair. These girls were probably just more sexually mature than the boys who were characterizing them. They weren't going along with the stereotype of being nice, passive girls sexually, so they took a lot of heat for just being different. But even though many of the boys put them down at school, we would go over to their houses after school, confirming the old double standard again. It seems likely that having their sexuality stigmatized at that time may have inhibited them sexually as adults. I hope not, for their sake.

The Madonna-Whore Dichotomy

The issues surrounding women's sexual assertiveness come into focus in what is commonly called the Madonna-whore dichotomy. The paradox here is that a man may crave a woman who seems virginal: innocent, aloof from sex, concerned only about motherhood and domestic issues. At the same time, he also wants a woman who is passionate, expressive, and very responsive about her sexuality. Obviously, there is a conflict. If the woman tries to meet one set of expectations, she finds herself clashing with the other set. When she tries to be sexually assertive and expresses her sexual desires, she is criticized for not being more Madonna-like; if she represses her sexuality, then she is accused of being frigid. It's a no-win situation.

Many women avoid this double bind by simply shutting down their sexuality altogether. They may dress and act in a way that minimizes their sexuality. They may fulfill their need for touching and loving through their children or by emotionally eating. If they eat to mask their emotions to cope with their situation, another problem arises: their weight becomes an issue that ends up blocking their sexuality. So many women and men I have seen tend to repress their sexuality once they find themselves in a committed relationship. They don't pay as much attention to the way they look and dress. They seem to be less concerned about their sexual appearance because they have a mate. They may not want to appear attractive to others so as not to create conflict with their commitment to monogamy. This process of shutting down one's sexuality generally occurs unconsciously.

The husband in this situation may go outside the marriage and have an affair to get his sexual needs met by way of a "whore-like" woman; i.e., a woman who enjoys sex. He then has his "Madonna" at home and "whore" outside the house.

This sort of arrangement was tacitly accepted and even encouraged during Victorian times. It still occurs today, but it is by no means accepted because it creates a great deal of pain and turmoil when the wife discovers what is going on. The acknowledgment of the affair is often the catalyst for divorce (though it is not generally its true cause).

This Madonna-whore syndrome surfaces in many relationships when the woman becomes pregnant or soon after the first child is born. Once she is a mother, she is no longer a sexual person in some men's view—and in the view of some women, too. This may be one of the contributing factors in the decline of sexual frequency during pregnancy or once a child is born. It might also account for the fact that some men have affairs at this point in the marriage. They can't see their wives as sexual beings now that their wives have become Madonnas.

The problem is that a woman just can't turn off her sexuality and all that entails when she is out in the world, and then all of sudden, turn her sexuality on like a light switch when she gets home. Sexuality isn't something you can compartmentalize. An individual's sexuality must be allowed to be free and flourish. Now, don't get me wrong, I am not talking about acting out sexually in terms of behavior. There are places and situations where appropriateness needs to be considered. Our sexuality involves so much more than just behavior.

When someone is newly single after being in a long-term relationship, they often want to be more attractive to the opposite sex and change the way they look and the way they live their life. They might lose weight, purchase different, more revealing clothing, and maybe buy a different, sexier car. These changes usually occur because they want to get their sexuality back. It's sad that they can't seem to maintain being sexy within a committed relationship. They have to be into the chase in order to be attractive.

Sexual Assertiveness

If the woman is sexually assertive, the man may become sexually passive. What effect does this role reversal have on him? The whole idea of a male being passive, in whatever context, is still culturally unacceptable. It goes against our stereotypical concept of manliness.

When a man becomes passive, his self-esteem and self-image may become deflated. But most important, it puts him in a vulnerable position. He is not in control, sexually speaking. For many men—particularly for those who are not confident about their own sexuality—it is very frightening not to be in control of what is happening sexually—unless it's part of some type of consensual sexual arrangement like bondage and dominance.

A cycle begins. When the man becomes sexually passive, his sexual self-esteem goes downhill. The lower his self-esteem, the harder and more risky it is for him to become the initiator of sex. He remains sexually passive—and the cycle perpetuates.

There is also a physiological component within the process. Studies of human males and lower primates under various conditions suggest a relationship between male testosterone secretion and certain psychological states. Low self-esteem, depression, humiliation, and rejection are all associated with a dramatically lowered testosterone level. With a lower testosterone level, the male's ability to be aggressive is inhibited; also, his sexual desire is reduced.

If you are a man caught in this cycle, it is vital that you break out. You can do this by developing higher self-esteem and confidence outside of the sexual relationship in which you feel that you have to be the aggressor. This can be done by becoming a part of some type of group or organization where you can get social support and validation. Being involved in some type of activity or sport can also help with developing self-esteem and confidence. If you don't do this, you are setting yourself up for failure.

A classic example of this cycle occurs when a newly divorced or separated man tries to establish a new relationship with a woman. His confidence is very shaky. He has left the shelter of a long-term marriage or relationship and now finds himself out in the cold, frightening, singles world. He might also be suffering from a sense of failure due to the breakup of his marriage or relationship. Clearly, his confidence is at a low ebb.

Where does he go to meet a woman? In the past, it used to be the local singles bar. For some men, this still may be the case, but for the majority today, dating sites on the Internet have replaced the singles bar. Both situations can be very intimidating places for a man who doesn't have much confidence sexually. To operate in the bar scene or on the Internet requires a good sense of self and an ability to aggressively pursue women. Even with those attributes, the experience can be disappointing, and often initiating relationships in these contexts can leave a man feeling worse than before he attempted to meet women. Women can, of course, have the same type of experience and emotions.

The behavior styles of being aggressive or passive can deaden sexual pleasure. Who would want to be in bed with a lover who is aggressive? This lover only cares about what he wants and is insensitive to his partner's emotions or desires and is always pushing his sexual agenda. Being aggressive in bed is like saying, "Come here, woman, and have sex with me. I don't care if you want to or not." On the other hand, who would want to have a sexual partner who is very passive? How boring. They just go along with what their partner wants and don't express any of their own desires. It's as if their body is there, but not their spirit.

What behavior style works in creating a healthy and fulfilling sexual relationship? The answer is being assertive. Assertiveness is saying what you want, but without the expectation that you will always get what you want. It means taking into consideration how your lover feels about your desire.

It is easier for men to make the transition to assertiveness because assertiveness doesn't altogether clash with our culture's concept of masculinity. However, for men who have been accustomed to getting their own way, the switch to the assertive stance can be difficult and threatening because it brings with it the possibility of losing control.

For those men who have been sexually passive, the switch to assertive behavior is perhaps more difficult. They have been accustomed to playing it safe with women, taking few risks. Sometimes, though, in trying to be more assertive, a passive man becomes aggressive because of built-up resentments acquired in his experience of being passive for so long.

The Effects of a Woman's Choices in Sexual Initiation

For women who have been traditionally passive in sexual relationships, the transition to assertiveness is very difficult. Years of unresolved and unconscious resentment may have accumulated. This may surface as a woman becomes assertive, leading to critical and demanding behavior, for which she may feel she will be judged. If she stumbles in her first inexpert attempts at self-assertion, she may feel guilty and return to the safety of passivity. Even women who are naturally sexually assertive run the risk of being judged as cheap or slutty by others in their community or by their partners.

Often, when I suggest to a woman that she make the first move by asking a man out to lunch or to meet him for a drink after work, she is afraid that he might feel threatened by her role reversal. This is also a concern in the context of the bedroom. A man may talk and fantasize about wanting his partner to be sexually assertive and initiate the lovemaking, but when she does, he may feel threatened and anxious.

Given these realities, the sexually assertive woman has to make a choice. Does she go back to being passive, waiting for her smartphone to ring or for an e-mail or text, allowing her lover to dictate the sexual agenda? If she does, she takes care of his insecurities and his need to be in control. She protects him from having to relate to an equal adult. This choice is supported by many of our cultural values. But what is the cost to the woman psychologically? The cost is resentment, low self-esteem, and the sense of not being in charge of her own life—i.e., being a child psychologically.

A little sexual assertiveness can help you see if the man you are involved with is one with whom you can form a long-term relationship—assuming that is your intention. You will probably have some lonely times, but I believe it is better to accept the loneliness than to damage your self-esteem to humor an insecure man.

When I ask couples whether they want sexual initiation to be mutual, they say yes. But what I find in reality is that this seldom happens. It's often the man who initiates sex in the beginning of a couple's relationship; as they age, his partner may start to initiate more often. The key is for the couple to be flexible concerning sexual initiation, as opposed to establishing some rigid pattern between them and becoming boring and predictable.

Making Your Sexual Needs Understood

One major problem couples have when it comes to initiating sex is clear communication. Often, they signal their desire to be sexual through a sort of code or by the use of innuendo. Perhaps one of them says, "I think I'll go upstairs and take a shower." Now this could mean that the person wants to get clean because they feel dirty, or it could mean that they are going to get clean because they want to have sex. How is their partner to know? It's all guesswork. Their partner might respond: "I'll be there in a few minutes." This could be interpreted as a yes to being sexual or as a statement that their partner is tired and just wants to go to sleep.

The stereotypical response of the woman who isn't interested in being sexual is, "I have a headache." Of course, the man could answer by saying, "Well, take some aspirin and I'll wait 20 minutes." However, what the woman is probably really trying to convey is a flat no to sex. But who knows?

To avoid disappointment, frustration, or hurt when asserting a sexual interest, you need to communicate clearly, which means being specific about what you want. Express yourself in such a way that your partner knows exactly what you have in mind. You don't have to be crude, unless that is something that you and your partner like. Also, clarity doesn't have to be unromantic or clinical. When you express yourself clearly, the odds of getting what you want increase greatly. There are still no guarantees, though—sorry!

Another benefit of clarity when it comes to sexual communication is that it prevents or reduces sexual assumptions. Since it is difficult for many couples in this culture to talk openly about sex, they tend to operate on unspoken assumptions. They assume they know what their partner likes or doesn't like, and what they want to do or don't want to do. Sometimes, their assumptions may be correct, other times, they may be way off base. A sexual relationship is too sensitive and emotional—and important—to leave to guesswork.

I once worked with a couple who both thought that their partner didn't enjoy oral sexual stimulation. They developed this assumption early in their relationship. By the time I saw them as patients, they had been married for eight years. One day in my office, they discovered through my questions that they had misinterpreted each other's reaction during one of their earliest sexual encounters. Because they had built the assumption into their subsequent lovemaking and had never communicated verbally about their preferences, they had lived together for almost a decade avoiding oral sex. They were both very surprised to discover that oral sex was high on each other's preference list. The lack of clear communication can distort a sexual relationship for a lifetime.

Structuring Time for Intimacy

Initiating sexual activity, even in a marital relationship, can be emotionally risky. As a way to minimize the emotional risk factor, some couples ritualize their initiation of sexual activity. They develop an understanding that at a certain time, they are supposed to become sexually involved—for example, Saturday night is sex night. Both partners have now succeeded in avoiding the emotional risk of initiating sex.

Unfortunately, eliminating risk also guarantees predictability. Without some spontaneity, sex becomes routine and boring. And if the prearranged time for sex rolls around and one of the partners isn't interested or is sick with a cold, the routine is disrupted. Maintaining this schedule would mean that if my partner were sick, I would have to wait a whole week until Saturday came around again. This kind of ritualization of sexual initiation feels too rigid and often has an adverse effect on sexual frequency.

In some situations, planning in advance or structuring time for a couple to be together intimately is necessary in order to maintain a long-term relationship. This is especially true if the couple has small children. Because couples think that their relationship is always going to be there, they sometimes take it for granted and put it on the back burner. Often, I hear this kind of dialogue in my office:

> "Honey, we don't spend enough time together."
> "Yes, we do. We spend all weekend together."
> "But we are with the kids at all their activities during the day and with our other couple friends in the evenings."
> "I would say we are together all the time."

This conversation identifies a typical problem facing many couples today: creating the time for their relationship. In today's busy world, trying to take care of all our relationships such as children, our jobs, family, and friends is a major task.

The one relationship we tend to neglect is the relationship with our spouse. Our culture's belief that marriage is "until death do us part" tends to set us up for taking the relationship for granted, creating an atmosphere of complacency.

Some people have the attitude that they got married so they wouldn't have to date anymore. I can understand not wanting to go through the hassle of meeting new people, but I wouldn't want to stop putting in the effort of making dates with my lover once the commitment to the relationship occurs. After all, what is a date but planning a time and place that is dedicated on your calendar to be with your spouse? Time for a couple to be alone so they may have intimate time together, whether an evening out or a weekend away without children, has to be set up in advance. It needs to be put on the couple's family calendar, along with the soccer matches and all the other events.

Couples need to create a boundary between all the incoming demands on their time and making time for their relationship. Without this boundary, their relationship will get lost among all the other activities. Commonly, when the very existence of the relationship is threatened, the couple becomes motivated to create the time and space to be together. Their relationship moves up to number one on their priority list. It's sad that the fear of losing the relationship is what motivates them. I would rather have their joy and pleasure in being together be the driving force to create a date for intimacy and romance.

When the time comes for the couple to be together, this does not necessarily have to be a sexual experience, unless that is something they both want to do. But it is important that they have time to be intimate, in the sense of being able to talk to one another about their inner thoughts and feelings and about the important things occurring in their lives. It is essential that they be able to communicate in this way without being interrupted by children walking in and begging for attention, or having to compete for attention with all the screens in their lives: cell phones, iPads, laptops, television, etc. This intimate time together on a regular basis is a necessary precursor to high-quality sexual activity in the bedroom—and a strong, lasting marriage.

Sex and Spontaneity

On the other end of the spectrum from those couples who ritualize their sexual involvement are those who feel that sexual initiation should always occur spontaneously. They believe that sex shouldn't require them to make plans ahead of time—it should just happen naturally, like spontaneous combustion. Sexual activity should just happen whenever the urge hits, no matter when or where.

Sexual spontaneity is great, and it happens a great deal when couples are young and in their twenties with a single lifestyle. There's nothing wrong with spontaneity—on the contrary! But for busy people and couples with children, spontaneity as a prerequisite for sex doesn't always work. It is hard to be spontaneous with children running in and out of the bedroom—or any other room, for that matter. Somehow, it seems that children have an intuitive sense of when their parents are being sexual, and they start crying or come and say hello at that very moment.

The only time that many couples with children can truly be spontaneous is when they are on a vacation without the children, staying in a hotel or resort. There, all they have is a room, a bed, and a television— which, hopefully, is off. In this sort of environment, spontaneous sexual combustion is much more likely to take place.

Why Do We Initiate Sex in the First Place?

Often, when I'm working with a person who has a lack of interest in sex, the issue of sexual initiation is a concern as well. It is not difficult to see why sexual interest and the ability to initiate sex are related. But just how are they related? What motivates a person to initiate sexual activity?

When I ask patients or students what impels them to have sex, usually they say, "I just feel like it," or, "It happens when I'm in the mood." They regard initiation as something you just don't think about—you just do it, kind of like the Nike ad. But when someone isn't initiating or participating sexually, then it becomes something we must look at closely.

The idea that sexual initiation is unpremeditated probably goes back to the formative period of the sexual relationship. In the beginning, the desire for sexual activity isn't an issue; it's just a matter of when and where. At this phase, interest is primarily physiologically based. Desire is driven by hormonal and biochemical agents. Testosterone, serotonin, oxytocin, and dopamine are operating at full blast on the brain. Psychologically, one or both partners are turned on sexually by the excitement, mystery, and newness of their developing relationship.

Anyone who has been in a long-term relationship knows that after a time, the novelty of the other person's body wears off. Both partners may still be quite attracted to each other physically, but perhaps there isn't the same, almost instantaneous response to seeing each other naked. You also sleep with that person every night, whereas before, there was a greater urgency because you might not seem them for a week or more. This is a normal pattern in long-term relationships.

But a problem arises if the couple's motivation for sex is limited to physiology—in other words, if they don't initiate or participate in sexual activity unless they are feeling "horny" or sexually aroused. Gradually, their relationship changes, to the point where they only feel the physiological urge perhaps twice a month. Their sexual frequency becomes limited to the infrequent times during which their hormone levels are at the right level to influence sexual desire.

Now, there is nothing wrong with initiating sex when the physiological urge motivates you; the problem is limiting your sexual expression to those times only. If your motivation to initiate sex is purely biological, then you are going to miss many opportunities to be sexual with your partner. What I propose to couples who find themselves in this predicament is that they add psychological motivators, which are not dependent on hormones, to their criteria for arousal.

The Two Psychological Motivators for Sexual Initiation

The Pleasure Principle

The first of these psychological motivators is the old Freudian pleasure principle. Simply put, this states that we keep on doing things from which we derive pleasure. If right at this moment your partner were to suggest that you both go out for ice cream, then, if you like ice cream and are not on a diet, you probably would say, "That sounds good—let's go!"

This same principle holds true for sex. If I think about making love to my wife, it usually equates with pleasure because that's what I experienced the last time we were involved sexually. Why wouldn't I want to experience that pleasure again? Pleasure has a carry-over effect.

People will go through a great deal of effort to reenact the pleasure of their previous experiences. One example is what people go through to experience the thrill and pleasure of downhill skiing or snowboarding. People say to me, "How can you go through all the hassle to go skiing? It's so cold, and you have to use chains on your tires to drive up to the hill. Then there are all the lines you have to wait in—and it's expensive." This is all true, and the answer is because it's so much fun and there is such a pleasurable rush to being up on the hill that it seems worth the hassle. The same can be said for what it takes some couples to be intimate.

The Gift of Love

The second psychological motivator derives from the fundamental symbolic meaning of sexual interaction in a loving relationship. Sex ideally represents the expression of the love between a couple. It is a gift of love, a way to bond or connect in a very intimate way. Of course, sexual expression doesn't always represent a loving expression; it can be a purely physical act done for self-pleasure, or, in worst - case scenarios, a weapon of power and control. As singer Tina Turner said in a hit song, "What's love got to do with it?" But for most couples in this Western culture, sexual intercourse represents the primary way to express their love for one another.

One example of a gift of love is oral sex. This form of sexual pleasure is a pure gift to one's lover because usually the pleasure for the giver is the pleasure they bestow upon their partner. This differs from intercourse, where there is more potential mutual physical sexual stimulation and pleasure.

These two motivators—being sexual because it felt pleasurable the last time, and because it is a way to express love—are ideally available to a couple every time they are in a sexually conducive environment. As much as the availability exists for these two motivators, they are both very vulnerable to inhibition.

What Inhibits Sexual Motivation?

What if your experience wasn't pleasant the last time you were involved sexually? What if it was frustrating, disappointing, or anxiety producing? You might be somewhat hesitant or cautious about initiating sexual activity. Perhaps the last time a man had intercourse, he lost his erection. If that happened, he may be less inclined to initiate sexual activity with his partner in order to avoid the embarrassment of feeling inadequate again. Or until he gets a prescription for erectile dysfunction medication.

As a therapist, I often see women who aren't interested in initiating sex with their partners because they do not experience orgasm. They receive pleasure from being close and being touched, but after a while, the frustration of not experiencing an orgasm outweighs this pleasure. Just as the carry-over effect can be a motivator, it can also be an inhibitor if the experience isn't pleasurable.

The second psychological motivator for initiating sexual activity—its meaning as an expression of love or as a way of bonding intimately—can also be inhibited. What if you and your spouse have been arguing all day and you have resentments that have not been resolved? You are not going to feel much like giving gifts of love when you go to bed at night.

So, while the two psychological motivators for sexual initiation are available to a couple every night, they can also be inhibited or blocked. When a couple goes to bed at night and they are both sexually available (i.e., neither is exhausted to the point of losing consciousness or physically sick) and one partner initiates sex and the other isn't interested, this is cause for concern. What concerns me more is not whether the couple is making love; rather, that the conditions in which lovemaking can occur don't exist between them—they haven't been nurtured and developed.

Generally, when this situation arises, the couple doesn't communicate much about the fact that they are emotionally distant. They both ignore the fact that something is wrong, kiss each other good night, and go to sleep.

I would like to invent a device that measures the level of emotional intimacy that exists between a couple. Let's call it an Intimacy Avoidance Detector. It would go over a couple's headboard in their bedroom—just like a smoke detector works in measuring whether smoke exists in a room. And we all know how irritating the sound is when that thing goes off. The same thing would happen with my device. The alarm would go off until the couple reestablished emotional intimacy.

Many couples who come to me don't see the many warning signals of a lack of emotional intimacy. Or maybe they just don't want to acknowledge their existence because it scares them to look at the issues. Either way, day after day goes by with both of them just going through the motions of everyday life, without making any real intimate connection with each other. They are just letting their relationship die right on the vine. They don't talk intimately, they are not very affectionate, and they're not very sexual. They are simply roommates. If this condition lasts for very long, irreparable damage can occur to the lover part of the relationship.

When your partner initiates sexual activity, if you are interested, then say yes by either participating in your partner's advances or by asserting your own desires. Remember that sexual activity does not have to include sexual intercourse. If you are not interested in sexual involvement, I recommend saying no, except for maybe a kiss and hug good night.

Some people, instead of saying no, go through a struggle with each other. Women tend to be in the position to make a decision more often because the man usually is the one making the advances. The struggle goes something like this:

"Honey, let's make love."
"No, I don't feel like it."
"Oh, come on, honey, it would be fun."
"No, I'm tired."
"Aww, come on."
"Okay. If that's what will make you happy."

This struggle can have very destructive consequences on the couple's communication specifically and their sexual relationship in general. This is a perfect example of where the female partner's sexual boundaries are not respected. She isn't respecting herself by participating sexually when she doesn't want to. The emotional outcome from her sexual participation under these circumstances will be resentment. After a while, she may start to hate being sexual with her partner because it represents a context in which she loses herself. She is in a psychological prison. It's not that she truly hates sex, just the context where saying no is not respected by her partner and herself.

Another consequence of this sexual struggle is that the female partner's credibility becomes questionable, at least within the sexual context. The initiator doesn't know what to believe when it comes to the other's sexual interest. Even when their partner does say yes, there will still be a question. This wondering—a mental activity—will get in the way of deep physical involvement because instead of enjoying to its fullest what is happening sexually, doubt will creep in. So, if you want to be sexual, say yes; if not, say no, and stick to it. It's that simple.

What To Do When Your Desires Aren't Clear

Our sexual desires are not always clear. Most of the time, I find myself in what I call the "gray zone." I am neither sexually turned on nor totally turned off. I am just neutral. Many of my patients, when approached by their lovers while in this neutral sexual state, will say no, saying they aren't in the mood.

What does it mean to be in a sexual mood? Does this mean that you have to be sexually aroused? I think for many people, the answer is yes. In order for many people to be sexually involved, they feel they must be sexually aroused at the outset. This belief is extremely limiting to a couple's sexual frequency and the amount of sexual pleasure in their life. An alternative belief would be to **lend yourself to the experience** when you are feeling sexually neutral or in the gray zone.

Most people don't live in what I would call a sexually erotic environment. I think that Hawaii, for example, can be a sexually erotic environment. What I mean by an erotic environment is a place where it's easy to relax and there isn't an overload of external stimulation that can cause stress. Instead, the external stimulation activates the senses in ways that cause a person to relax. When you get to Hawaii or some other exotic location, the smells of the flowers, the warmth of the sun, the visual beauty of the colors of the sea, sky, and land, the feel of the trade winds, and the sound of the surf can move you from the mainland into a place of relaxation—a major precursor to great sex. Sometimes, it might take a few days for a person from the city to make this transformation, but once he or she does, it's awesome.

Unfortunately, most of us don't live in one of these environments—we might only vacation there occasionally. Where we live is often full of external stressors such as traffic, street noise, crowds of people, and the biggest stressor of all, work.

Let's say that after working all day and living in such an environment for the past eight hours, I come home and my wife asserts herself by saying, "Dan, let's go in the bedroom and fool around." At that moment, sex may be the last thing on my mind. (I know that might be hard to believe given what I do for a living, but it happens.) What is my answer? If I base my response on the idea that I have to be sexually aroused in the moment, then my answer will be, "No, honey, I'm not in the mood." I might be thinking about the patients I saw earlier in the day. But if I base the answer on an attitude of openness, then I will say, "Sure, that sounds great, let's go upstairs." If I choose the second option, then I am lending myself to a sexual experience to see what happens. And, of course, once I do that, I stop thinking about all the things that have been causing me stress, and I start thinking about how good my wife looks and how much pleasure I feel when she is touching and kissing me in such a loving way.

In lending myself to the sexual experience, I gain an important understanding: just because I become sexually involved doesn't necessarily mean that I am going all the way to having intercourse or an orgasm. As I said in the previous chapter, just because I am getting on the train in San Francisco doesn't necessarily mean that I am going to New York. Who knows? I might want to stop in Reno for the night. If there is pressure applied either by my partner or by myself to go all the way sexually, then I won't want to be involved because I may only want to just hold and touch her and not have intercourse. If there is no pressure, then I will often want to go all the way.

Does this mean that we can't say no to our partner's sexual advances? We are drawing an important distinction here—especially for women. Remember, in the Victorian period, sex was one of the wifely duties. A woman couldn't refuse and still be a good wife. But men have difficulty with this issue as well. We're told a "real man" always wants sex and is always ready to have it. So, if a man were to say no, he wouldn't be living up to this false image of masculinity.

If a woman or a man is involved sexually without really wanting to be involved, then that person will consciously or unconsciously resent what is happening. This resentment will build and collect over time and contaminate the couple's relationship to the point that one or both partners will turn off to sex and eventually to the marriage as well. What may seem like a gift now may be a curse in the long run. Giving sexually is only a gift if no resentment is involved. If resentment is involved, then the gift is very expensive, emotionally speaking.

The bottom line is if you're feeling neutral, you might try lending yourself to the experience. But if you definitely do not want to participate, just say no.

The Fear of Rejection

For everyone—teenagers or adults, married people or people living together, or singles dating—sexual initiation raises the fear of rejection. And for many of us, this fear gets in the way of initiating sexual activity. The lower an individual's confidence or self-esteem, the more this becomes an issue.

To be turned down for sex, even in marriage, is a blow to one's ego or pride. To protect ourselves, we wait for the other person to make the first move. Fear of rejection is particularly anxiety producing for men because they are usually expected to make the first move and most often run the risk of being turned down.

Women also have a fear of rejection and may take their lover's lack of interest in them as a form of passive rejection. They may become insecure about their appearance or their ability as a lover. This happens most frequently when their male partner is in the age range of 40 and beyond. The men always seem too tired for sex, or they drink too much and fall asleep in front of the television.

The initiation discussion reminds me of my first dating experiences. As a man, I was expected to ask the girl out for a date. I had to make that phone call. This, in a way, was the beginning of my sexual initiation experience. By asking that girl for a date, I was putting my neck on the chopping block. Without knowing it, she had the power to decide my worth relative to the opposite sex—I gave her that power. My ego and self-esteem as a lover hung in the balance.

If she said no to going out with me, I believed that she was rejecting me, and being rejected really hurt and then turned to anger. If she said yes, then I kept my head and was spared the "blade of rejection." My mother never had to ask me what the girl said. If she said yes, then I would be running around asking my mother if there was anything I could do to help her, but if the girl said no, I got mad, slamming doors and turning my stereo up loud.

When a girl said no to a date, she never said why, just no. I went away feeling worthless. My parent may have told me that maybe her parents didn't want her dating, but, of course, I thought it was all about me in a negative way. I am sure that girls feel rejected if boys don't ask them out for a date. I know my own daughters felt that way if they weren't asked to dance when they went to a school dance.

My desire to initiate sexual activity with girls and the risk of personal rejection continued through high school and my college experience. It wasn't until I was in my mid-twenties and going to clubs that I started to examine this concept of personal rejection and sexual initiation within the singles adult dating world.

If I went to a party or club and asked a woman to dance and she said no, was she rejecting me? What if I asked another woman for her phone number and she said no? Was she rejecting me? Or how about if I asked another woman to go home with me for some late-night activity and she said no, was she rejecting me? I discovered the answer to all of these questions was no.

Here's why. In the situation described above, what the woman was saying no to was what/wanted, my personal agenda. Everyone in the singles world has an agenda of some kind. They want something. It could be to get married, to have a one-night stand, or maybe just have a dance and nothing more. In the singles world, interactions happen so fast that the women I encountered couldn't possibly have gotten to know me on any meaningful level. The women I interacted with didn't know my personal values, personality traits, or interests, since it takes time to get to know someone.

In today's dating environment, things have changed. With so many people meeting via the Internet, potential dates know a lot more information about a person before they ever meet them in real time. But even in today's high-speed Internet–dating world, the knowledge shared is still somewhat superficial. It takes time and real interaction to really get to know what someone is really like. Most single encounters don't involve that kind of time.

Simply put, the women I encountered with my agenda or desires didn't really know enough about me to reject me as a person. What they were saying no to was what I wanted, not me, because they didn't really know me well enough to reject me. It wasn't personal. I was disappointed because

I wasn't getting what I wanted—that is part of adult life. We don't always get what we want. Being disappointed is very different from being rejected, because the latter can really hurt emotionally and have a devastating impact on an individual's sexual self-esteem. Once I understood this distinction, sexual initiation was much less intimidating than before. I could express my desires to any woman without the fear of rejection because she couldn't reject me; she didn't know me.

So far, I have only talked about the fear of rejection in the context of the singles world. Let's look at rejection in a long-term relationship such as marriage. You would think that once a couple made a long-term commitment to each other that the issue of sexual rejection wouldn't be an issue, but it still exists.

Suppose that I am being assertive. I clearly express to my wife my desire to have sex with her and she says, "No, not tonight, Dan. I'm just too tired." Is she rejecting me sexually? Again, the answer is no.

In this case, my wife isn't rejecting me; she is just saying no to what I want. We have conflicting agendas: I want to make love, but she wants to sleep. Both agendas are legitimate, but they're in conflict with each other. If I understand the difference between rejection and disappointment, I don't react with the emotions of hurt and anger. I just feel the frustration of not getting what I want in the moment.

Men who take disappointment as rejection feel really hurt and angry. They often act out these emotions by pouting, giving dirty looks, slamming doors, or giving the silent treatment. None of these forms of communication are attractive or erotic; on the contrary, they turn their partner off even further to participating in any sexual interaction. They also impede any real effective communication.

When I ask men why they perceive that their wife is sexually rejecting them, I try to get them to tell me specifically what she is rejecting about them by asking questions: "Is she rejecting the way you look? Is it the way you make love? Is it the way you approach her to have sex?" Usually they respond, "I don't know; she is just rejecting me."

For my wife to reject me sexually, she would have to say something like, "No, not tonight or ever, Dan, because you are a sexual pervert, fat, and ugly, and one of the most disgusting human beings I've ever met!" Now, that's personal rejection.

When I am sexually disappointed, instead of acting out my frustration in a way that turns my lover off, I want to explore her resistance to being sexually involved. I am not trying to pressure her to have sex; I just want to find out what's in the way. When I do this, it tells her that I care about her as a person and that she just isn't an object for my sexual satisfaction. She may feel resistant because she doesn't feel emotionally close enough to make love. Perhaps she is still angry about something I said or did earlier in the day. Maybe the resistance has nothing to do with me personally; it might be that she is feeling very anxious about something going on with her work situation. Maybe she is feeling inadequate about her sexual abilities, and is afraid to be sexually involved. In all these cases, it has little to do with the sexual rejection of me as her lover.

If her resistance is related to me, then I want to explore how to remove the barrier to being sexually intimate by using the effective communication techniques as described in my book, *Creating the Intimate Connection*.(2) Especially critical is effective listening to whatever is emotionally blocking my wife from being sexually involved. We may not make love that night, but at least we are emotionally close enough if we choose to be sexual the following day.

I hope that with an understanding of the difference between sexual rejection and disappointment, it will be easier for you to assert yourself sexually in whatever kind of personal relationship you may be involved.

Creating a Context for Intimacy

The last aspect of sexual initiation I would like to address involves setting the scene; that is, sexuality beyond what you do physically in bed. In today's Internet world, there is very little modeling for young men and women on what it means to create a romantic, sensual atmosphere in which sex can occur. For some, this may seem old-fashioned, but when you take the romance, and especially the sensuality, out of the sexual context, you are just left with sex—and that can get pretty limited and boring.

When adults used to date as opposed to "hooking up," setting the scene was imperative. The goal was to make the other person want to be with you in an intimate way. For men, the idea often was to make the conquest, and their goal-oriented sexual world may have included a "seduction den." Sexual seduction requires lots of effort, advance planning, and preparation. Nothing was spontaneous.

When I was single and had a date with a woman I really cared about, I would try to make sure that everything went smoothly. I made reservations at a special romantic restaurant, including the right table with the best location where it wasn't noisy so you could hear each other talk. I cleaned my car and made sure that my house, bedroom, and bathroom were also clean and neat. I chose appropriate clothes for the evening. Once we were back at my place, I lit a fire and some candles, and put on some mellow background music. The scene was set.

Somehow, I think that creating this type of environment and experience may have been lost with the members of Gen Y and beyond. Today, many couples just hook up and don't really date in the traditional way that I just described. If they don't create this type of sexual experience when they are going out, they certainly are not going to do it when they are in a marital relationship. There is no precedent established to carry on after they say "I do."

When I was dating, why did I put so much energy and effort into trying to make the evening special? One goal was to get my date in a sexy and romantic mood so that she would feel comfortable and relaxed and would want to go to bed with me. Yes, I had a very self-centered interest, but not at her emotional expense. Another goal was to show her how much I cared about her by making such an effort. If I were going over to a woman's house for dinner, I might experience the same type of evening because she would reciprocate with the same amount of effort.

There is nothing wrong with any of this type of behavior. But a problem may occur when the "goal" has been achieved—when the conquest has been made or the commitment to the relationship has been established. The mountain has been climbed. Now what? The motivation to create a romantic or erotic atmosphere is no longer present. The attitude becomes "Let's just get it on and jump into the sack. Let's stop wasting our time with this preliminary stuff." This attitude opens the door to complacency and to taking one's significant other for granted. It is particularly dangerous for couples who have been married for a few years.

I'm not saying that every time you plan to be sexually involved with your lover or spouse you have to spend hours creating a romantic mood and environment. But you should consider doing so more than twice a year—at the very least on your anniversary and on Valentine's Day!

Creating a romantic mood is especially important for couples with small children. It's hard to put yourself into a lover's frame of mind when you have diapers and kids' toys everywhere. It becomes essential for the couple to create some kind of refuge within their house, where they can be alone. What is even more important than having a refuge is having a lover's consciousness: looking at each other as a woman and man, as opposed to just a wife and husband or mother and father.

Keeping the Fires of Passion Alive in a Long-Term Relationship

How can a couple stop taking their sexual relationship for granted, once the goal of the conquest has been achieved and they have committed to stay together? They need some type of motivation to take the place of getting the person to be with them. They are now with their lover every night.

I went through a personal journey of discovering how to maintain sexual attraction throughout the course of a committed relationship. It was after I was married and had children that the idea of maintaining a lover's consciousness became a high priority in my life. My patients and attendees at my seminars told me that my ideas sounded great on paper, but with the reality of marriage and children, I must see that they were too idealistic to be practical. They wanted me to agree with them that marriage and children inevitably drive your love life down the tubes. What more could one expect? That's just the way it is.

After being married for a long time and having children who are now adults themselves, my experience has taught me is that it is possible to maintain a high degree of romance and intimacy in a long-term relationship. The key is motivation and the ability to create this kind of relationship in the context of marriage. A couple needs to have the skills and beliefs that foster intimacy. They might be motivated, but without the skill set, they will become frustrated and lose the motivation to continue.

Another key variable is that both individuals in the relationship must have the same desire and motivation to keep their relationship intimate and vital. If one partner is trying and the other isn't, the relationship will eventually end. As the old saying goes, "It takes two to make a marriage work."

Creating a Sexual Ambience

I learned valuable lessons in creating a romantic sexual atmosphere from a roommate I had when I was 26 and single. I don't believe that he knew at the time that I was learning from him, but in hindsight, I found out a great deal. When I was looking for a roommate, I wanted someone who might give me access to meeting women. He managed a large restaurant with lots of female waitstaff, so I thought that he would be a great contact person for meeting women. He also had a great stereo system and good food. He was an expert at creating a sexual ambience. When my roommate first moved into his bedroom in my house, he started decorating his bedroom in the way I would decorate a living room. He put in attractive, comfortable chairs, a fish tank, ferns, a small stereo, and he hung decorative rugs on the wall. He created a very warm and sensual environment to hang out in and just relax. My bedroom down the hall was the complete opposite. I had just a bed, a dresser, a mirror, and a poster on the wall. My room lacked any warmth and sensuality. It felt more like a motel room than a living space.

Not surprisingly, the women my roommate knew did not want to hang out in my room. I had to hear them having a good time. It was a very frustrating experience.

My plan to meet women backfired, but I did learn a valuable lesson. At that time, I was waiting for a woman who would come into my life and decorate my room and the rest of the house. I was waiting for a woman to complete me with her femininity. My personality had very little sensuality or softness to it, and this lack was expressed in the way I interacted with women. When a woman I was dating tried to fill this void in my makeup, I would feel uncomfortable. It felt like she was acting like my mother. Because of their efforts, I tended to push these women away. None of this was done consciously, but I could only see the pattern later when I looked back on this period of my life. The women I was attracted to didn't want to be with me because they sensed that I was looking to them to complete me, and they wanted no part of that responsibility. The result was that I didn't have a serious relationship for at least two years.

My breakthrough came when I realized that I needed to take responsibility to fill that void in myself, as my roommate had done for himself, if I wanted to be sexually attractive to women who weren't codependent. I needed to develop the feminine side of my own personality, so that I was balanced in my gender makeup. I needed to decorate my own house and stop waiting for a woman to do it for me. This change wasn't just about decorating my house, but many other aspects of my life. I learned to cook, clean, shop, and buy my own clothes—everything that my mother did for all the males in my family. I reached the point where I didn't need a woman to exist. I was no longer dependent.

This concept of being a male who is self-sufficient in all areas of his life wasn't modeled for me growing up in the 1950s and 1960s. I never saw my father involved in anything that might be considered feminine. By the mid-1970s, gender roles were changing all around me, and I needed to change as well to stay current with the times if I wanted a relationship that lasted.

Sexuality Beyond the Bedroom

My roommate also taught me another lesson, which had to do with the shape my body was in and the type of clothes I wore. At that age, I didn't really pay attention to those things. I played lots of tennis and skied. I could eat whatever I wanted and not worry about my calorie intake. Those were the days.

Of course, a woman's physical body shape made a big difference to me. Men were always checking women out with that "meat market" mentality. I wasn't exempt from that type of mindset. I had never heard about women looking at men in the same way. Of course they did; I just didn't know about it.

My roommate told me that women also like to look, and that they are aroused by the way a man is physically built. They like men with cute rear ends and flat stomachs, although they may not be as vocal about their preferences when compared to men. It hasn't really been until the last 20 years or so that men acquired the same concern.

With the insight that women are turned on by a man's physical appearance, I started running and playing tennis differently. At first, my motivation to run wasn't about health, it was more about appearing sexy. Later, it became about my general health. My approach to tennis changed from being about just trying to win a tournament, to trying to stay in better physical shape. This would help my sexual self-esteem and my general health. So, tennis became a win-win opportunity for me because even if I didn't win the match, I still walked off the court feeling improved physically and didn't leave feeling like a total loser.

I don't advocate extremes of self-indulgence and narcissism; I believe that each person can find a happy medium between physical narcissism and being a pot-bellied couch potato. Some people take their physical appearance to an extreme where they are constantly obsessing about how they look, constantly working out in the gym to the point that it's about all they do with their free time.

When I was in my twenties, I didn't much care how my clothes looked when I went out on a date, as long as what I wore was clean and neat. I had come out of the 1960s counterculture, so I had no regard for fashion, unless it was antifashion. I did pay attention to how my date was dressed, though, and I soon realized that I had a double standard when it came to clothes.

At this time, I also became aware of the role that my clothes played in terms of my sexuality. When I was dating, my mother always told me how to dress, but, of course, I would resent her unsolicited advice. I would rebel and do the opposite and resist her efforts at trying to influence my fashion choices, even if they were the right choices at that time. But I could receive the information from a peer.

When I put on my first pair of Calvin Klein designer jeans, I soon realized that I was making a sexual statement. How I dressed when I went out on a date started to make a big difference. I started to invest in having a fashionable wardrobe, as opposed to trying to get by with the cheapest clothes that I could find. In physical and metaphorical terms, I tossed out my faded Levi's with their holes and patches. After all, it was 1976, and the times were changing; that meant it was time for me to change my attitude.

Treating Love as Though It Matters

The change in the way I dressed was illustrated when I would go out on a date with someone. I became conscious of the casual clothes I chose to wear. I wanted to make myself attractive to women. After I was married, I became aware of a trap that many married men fall into. When I went to work, I wore the nicest clothes I owned. I wanted to dress for success. When I went out to a show or dinner with my wife, I didn't pay as much attention to my clothes as I did when we were dating. I just wanted to be comfortable. While there's nothing wrong with comfort, in my case, it represented the great enemy of a lover relationship—complacency—creeping in. This isn't just about clothes, but the approach to the relationship in general.

Why is it that once we are married or in a committed relationship, we lose this concern? We begin to think that the marriage is forever, and that our spouse will always be there, no matter what. It's the attitude of "until death do us part" having its effect on our behavior. Once we begin to take our partner for granted, we are guaranteeing trouble for the relationship.

It is not uncommon for someone who is separated and not interested in getting back with their spouse (or at least not right away) to make personal changes, all having to do with their sexuality—losing weight, perhaps making a trip to a plastic surgeon, getting a different wardrobe, maybe buying a new sports car. It's as if this person could not let his or her sexuality out within the marital context. Now that they are outside the marriage relationship, they want to regain their sexuality so they are more attractive to potential lovers.

Why do we have to be separated or single in order to keep our sexuality alive? Is it because we can't handle monogamy? Are we afraid that if we maintain an ongoing sexuality, we will attract the opposite sex and yield to temptation?

Men and women who downplay their sexuality by gaining weight or dressing less stylishly may be trying to control their relationship by subconsciously denying a basic part of their identity. If they can downplay their sexual appeal, then others won't come on to them and they will avoid any potential conflicts, at least externally. Of course, shutting their sexuality down doesn't help the intimacy level within their marriage. Perhaps they don't feel confident about the quality of the relationship or their own commitment to it. The more the relationship lacks in intimacy and love, the more this pattern takes over.

Whenever people try to control an intimate relationship in this way, their efforts often backfire and destroy the relationship. They trap themselves by denying their full sexual potential. And they deny their spouse a partner who is fully open to them on a sexual level. The marriage becomes a self-created prison, from which either party is glad to escape.

Making an effort to keep romance in your long-term relationship pays off handsomely. Romance, as well as being pleasant in and of itself, is a terrific relationship-builder. As Alan and Donna Brauer say in their book, *ESO*, "If you think romance is a waste of time, think again. Paying attention to romance will win your romantic partner's warm attention in return. Isn't that what you want?"(3)

Romance and sex are words that can naturally go together, but many couples today don't seem to make romance a priority in their daily lives, saving it for special occasions like Valentine's Day or their anniversary. The rest of the year, they ignore it. Sexuality has to do with the way we communicate, the way we deal with conflicts, and the way we spend time together. When you are with a lover, you are obviously not in bed all the time; you spend time together walking on the beach or having a picnic in the countryside, or sharing time together in some other way that you both enjoy. It is important to focus on being together, as opposed to the activity. I like to make the distinction between "be" versus "do." Romance and intimacy are more about the *being* together than what you are *doing*.

All of these situations are opportunities for romance and for nurturing the lover aspect of your relationship. None of this has to change just because a commitment has been made or because you are married.

Motivating Yourself to Love

The question remains, how do you motivate yourself to maintain a lover's consciousness in a long-term, intimate relationship? Couples are highly motivated to create romance and intimacy when they have the goal in mind of trying to get their lover in some kind of way. They might be trying to get a boyfriend or girlfriend, or to get a husband or wife, or they may just be trying to get their partner in bed with them to engage in a sexual experience. Once they have accomplished their goal, what will motivate them to keep treating their partner in a romantic, sexual way?

Often, when I see a couple who are separated, one of them is very motivated to get their spouse back. If it's the husband, he just doesn't send his wife one dozen roses, but three. He writes many cards or e-mails expressing his love for his spouse. The husband wants to initiate romantic dinners or weekend getaways to a romantic destination. Before the separation, none of this energy was apparent. Now, it's all happening with the goal of getting the spouse back, but what happens once he succeeds at achieving his goal? Does this energy disappear? His spouse may question his continued credibility because she can see that the motivation arises from desperation, rather than a true understanding of how to improve their relationship.

I tell the man if he wants my help in getting back with his spouse, he needs to change his approach. It's usually men who are in this position within the relationship, but occasionally a woman may also be trying to get her husband back. It's paradoxical: you can't "get" someone—they need to want to be with you. And you do that by making yourself more appealing. Coming on so strong out of nowhere is not appealing. It's overwhelming and usually a turn-off. On the other hand, acting in more ways that aren't pushy or aggressive allows the other spouse to choose to be with him or not. It's about being vulnerable and not trying to control someone so they say they love you.

When people come to me asking how to keep their relationship alive, I try to help them see the rewards that will come from exerting the extra energy it will take. Usually, if I tell them that they should do this because it will improve their relationship, they will hear the logic, but their motivation only lasts a short time; and then they go back to their old, complacent ways. It can't be an "I should," but instead it must be an "I want" to maintain motivation.

One of the great realizations I had when I pursued women as a single man was how much I enjoyed having a romantic experience with someone I cared about, and how much I enjoyed having and planning romantic dinners and weekends with a lover. I looked forward to sharing great food, beautiful nature, and wonderful sexual experiences together. What was not to like? It was wonderful.

Once I realized how enjoyable these experiences were, my motivation started to change from creating and initiating these types of romantic and intimate experiences for the woman I was with, to doing it for my own pleasure. It's not that the woman I was with didn't enjoy what was happening as well, but that wasn't my main motivation as it had been before.

The driving factor for cultivating your own lover's attitude must be your own pleasure. If you are merely trying to make your partner happy and see sex as an obligation, then your efforts will come to nothing. You will continue to make your partner happy if you put energy into your relationship because it makes you feel good. It's as simple as that.

A classic example of this concept is the way many people look at Valentine's Day. Some look at it as what they call a "Hallmark holiday" and dismiss its value. They see it as just a holiday created to sell flowers, cards, and chocolates. I think this attitude is sad because they don't see Valentine's Day as a celebration of the love between their lover and themselves. To them, it's just a day of expectations and obligation. For me, it's Christmas for lovers. I don't have to buy a card, roses, or chocolate. I want to because it's a great way to express and celebrate the joy of my intimate relationship. Hopefully, this celebrating occurs more than one day a year, and it will if you are motivated by your desire for pleasure and not obligation.

When I got married, I didn't want to stop dating a lover. I wanted to treat my wife as if she was still my lover. Just because we had a commitment to monogamy did not mean that I wanted that part of our relationship to change.

Many people don't believe it's possible to maintain being lovers—and I don't just mean having sex—in a long-term marriage. They think it's just a Hollywood fantasy. I have never shared that belief. I think it is possible, but it requires motivation and an understanding of what it takes to continue being lovers.

In the beginning of my career, I gave seminars to the public about marriage and intimacy even before I was married. At the end of the seminar, the attendees would ask questions. Often, the first question was whether I was married. I didn't wear a wedding ring, so they probably knew that I wasn't. When I told them I wasn't married, they would sometimes say, "Well, wait until you get married, because everything you say sounds good, but after you get married, you will see that the intimacy will fade away." I didn't agree with them because of what I knew about how to create emotional intimacy within a long-term relationship, but I felt that couldn't say anything to refute their claim since I wasn't married.

After I got married, I proudly wore my wedding ring when I gave seminars. At the end, participants didn't ask me if I was married, but instead they asked me if I had children. Again, they often expressed a negative, pessimistic attitude about maintaining intimacy when you have children. Of course, having children creates a greater challenge, but it's still possible if the desire and knowledge is present to have passion and a great sex life and to view your partner as a lover, rather than a roommate. After raising two wonderful daughters, I still hold this belief today.

A second motivation for nurturing your love relationship—and a very real one—is the fear of losing your lover and your relationship because of neglect. Often, the biggest symptom that your relationship is suffering is that your lover might end up having an affair. It is naive to think that your wife just takes care of the kids at home and that's all she cares about, especially if she works outside the home, or that your husband is too busy with work and he's just not the type of guy to have an affair. If you are not treating your spouse like a lover, then some very important emotional needs are not being fulfilled. The likelihood of an extramarital affair occurring increases dramatically, if either partner has much self-esteem. I know this sounds harsh, but that's the reality in today's world. According to one website, conservative estimates are that 65 percent of men and 55 percent of women in the United States will have an extramarital affair.(4)

Both motivations, one being the desire for the pleasure of intimacy and the other the fear of losing a relationship for maintaining an intimate relationship once a commitment is involved, arise from a core desire that I assume you have—the desire for a lover. If that is not what you want, if your relationship is just a game or a strategy for staving off abandonment fed from a core insecurity of being alone in the world, then you and your partner need to know that. But if you do, in fact, want a passionate, exciting, and pleasurable relationship, then you can have what you want—if you are willing to invest some time and effort in the ways we've considered in this chapter.

Sexual initiation is much more than what you do in the bedroom. It concerns how much you are willing to acknowledge your own and your partner's sexuality. You do this by understanding that you do not have to limit yourself to the rigid rules of initiation that society teaches us. You do it by recognizing that spontaneity sometimes needs a little assistance. You do it by learning to communicate honestly and openly about what you want sexually. You do it by remembering that the romance that makes any relationship exciting needs a bit of nurturing throughout the length of the relationship.

Works Cited

1. Parrott, Dr. Les. *Crazy Good Sex*. Grand Rapids, MI: Zondervan, 2009.
2. Beaver, Daniel. Creating the Intimate Connection: The Basics to Emotional Intimacy. San Diego: Cognella, 2010.
3. Brauer, Alan, & Brauer, Donna. *ESO: How You and Your Lover Can Give Each Other Hours of Extended Sexual Orgasms*. New York: Wellness Central, Hachette Book Group, 2001.
4. http://www.todayschristianwoman.com/articles/2008/september/why-affairs-happen.html

9

How Often is Normal?

Sexual Frequency Issues

When I trained as a sex therapist in the 1970s, the issue of sexual frequency wasn't presented as one of the basic sexual problems between couples. Today, sexual frequency issues seem to be the number one presenting problem with couples and individuals seeking my therapeutic help.

Author David Atkins states, "The number one sexual problem facing most couples is low or no sex or discrepancies in sexual desire between spouses. Studies have found that one in three women and one in seven men report low sexual desire. When one spouse pushes for sex while the other tries to avoid it at all cost, conflict, frustration and boredom will often happen in the relationship."(1)

So why was this issue not considered important 40 years ago, while today it has become a major concern? I believe it has something to do with a couple's lifestyle and how things have changed, including the increased pace of life today.

The commitment of many couples to work has increased greatly, to the point that the 40-hour workweek is no longer the norm in many professions. The amount of time people spend just commuting to their jobs cuts deeply into the time they have to spend with their partner. As I stated in Chapter Seven, work and sexual pleasure are natural enemies, and the more personal the commitment to work, the more inroads it makes into one's sexual life. With the recent economic downturn, people are working even more hours if they have a job, and if they are out of work, their anxiety about being unemployed also takes its toll on their intimate life.

It's true that many people are working longer hours than in the past, but we have been through hard economic times before, so why has this had such an impact on couple's sexual frequency? The reason is that the expectation for having an active sex life has changed. In the past, people's expectation regarding sexual frequency was lower. The baby boomers and subsequent generations expect sex, regardless of the physical and psychological conditions.

Consequently, many couples today find themselves in a state of cognitive dissonance between their expectations regarding sexual frequency and their reality—that they work a lot and are tired when they come home, especially by the time they are ready to go to sleep.

Cognitive dissonance simply means noise in the brain; an individual is in a state of psychological disharmony or conflict. People tend to react to this situation of internal conflict with the emotions of resentment, anger, and disappointment. These emotions don't foster erotic feelings, and thus shut down at least one partner's sexual desire.

As Atkins states, "When one spouse pushes for sex while the other tries to avoid it at all cost, conflict, frustration and boredom will often happen in the relationship. Often with inhibited desire of one spouse, the other spouse becomes pushy and resentful, which leads to lack of affection and closeness. The longer the couple avoids sexual contact it becomes harder to break the cycle. The longer they hold back from sexual contact, the more they tend to blame each other."(2) The blame game becomes a vicious circle, which can lead to very little sexual activity for both individuals.

The way to relieve the cognitive dissonance is to change an individual's sexual expectations to be more in line with their reality. If both partners work all day, either outside or inside the home, and they are both exhausted by the time they go to bed, then it isn't realistic to expect a sexual experience. It's not an optimal situation, but it is a common one, given the lifestyle many people lead in our society.

It's more about the quality than the quantity of sexual experiences. So during the workweek, sexual activity between a couple may be more of an exception, but they might want to plan for a great sexual experience for the weekend, preferably Saturday night when their energy level is higher. Having more energy will lead to better and more fulfilling sex.

So How Often Is Normal?

As a therapist, one of the questions I am most frequently asked is: "How often is it normal for a couple to make love? Is it once a week, every day, three times a day, or once a month?"

Of course, statistics seem to answer this question. But I am not going to cite those statistics here, because to do so would only serve to further concretize the assumptions that are built into the question. I try to stay away from any discussion about what is "normal." Who I am I to determine what is normal for a couple to be sexual with one another? I recommend that couples also ignore the statistics, since whatever statistics come to mind tend merely to be used as ammunition for debate.

A frequency problem exists not when a couple deviates from some statistical norm, but when there is a significant discrepancy between the desires of the two people—when, for example, one partner wants to make love once a week, while the other wants to do so once a month. Now, that's a frequency problem. If, on the other hand, both partners are content with being sexually involved once a month, then who is to say that they have a problem? Frequency is a problem when a conflict of sexual desires exists in the couple's relationship. It's a conflict that needs to be resolved; otherwise, this unresolved conflict will only continue to create resentment that will block sexual desire, which, in turn, makes the problem of frequency worse.

Sexual frequency statistics don't take into account the context in which a couple is interacting. In the beginning of a new relationship, sexual frequency is higher when compared to when the couple has a baby and then small children. Frequency will be quite different when the couple has been together for 15 years, as compared to when a couple enters the menopause years. So, to pick some statistical number that doesn't include the context of the marital relationship doesn't make sense.

Another reason that frequency is more of an issue than in the past is that it has become acceptable for women to want more sexual frequency within their marriage. As a result, they are less willing to accept a limited sex life than they might have been in the past.

This may be uncomfortable for husbands who are accustomed to being in the controlling position, at least as far as sexual initiation. They may perceive their wives' increased interest as pressure on them to perform, which, in turn, may intimidate them and cause them to become less interested in sex. The outcome, often, is reduced frequency.

Quality and Sexual Frequency

One of the primary bases for an active sexual relationship is the quality of the experience for the partners involved. Good quality usually means a high level of sexual pleasure. When the amount of sexual pleasure drops off for either partner, then that partner loses interest. That's when sexual frequency becomes a problem.

Generally, when I see couples with sexual frequency problems, one partner's sexual desire is really high, nearly insatiable, and the other's is almost nonexistent. The stereotype is that the woman in the relationship is the partner whose sexual desire is nonexistent. This may be true earlier in a marriage, but it can shift when men move into their forties and beyond. Their desire is often a lot lower, while their wife's desire increases.

Let's look at the case of Sue and Jack, in a stereotypical situation. Jack seems to always want to have sex, while Sue could take it or leave it. Like many couples who have the same problem, Sue and Jack follow a certain pattern, or scenario. It's as if they are following an unwritten script.

Usually, Jack and Sue wait to have sex until late at night, when the kids have gone to sleep, all their chores are done, and their favorite television shows are over. If it is a weekday, they have both worked all day. They are tired, if not exhausted. Still, they have to get up early and get the kids ready for school and get themselves ready to go to work. They can't sleep in and have a leisurely morning together in bed.

Despite these factors, when Sue and Jack get into bed together, Jack immediately wants to make love. In fact, from Sue's point of view, Jack's sex drive is insatiable—all he wants to do is have sex. The minute they are in bed together, his arm comes over to her and he starts touching her with the intent to have sex. She moves it away, saying that she is too tired to have sex, but he puts it back, hoping that she will give in to his desires.

Sue, in comparison to Jack, would probably like to have sex maybe once a month. Instead, he keeps touching or grabbing her in the same way he does every night, not paying attention to her resistance to being sexually involved. She feels pressure to have sex because she thinks,"If I don't have sex with him, he might go somewhere else. I do love him and he works so hard to support us. After, all, it's my wifely duty." You can hear the fear of abandonment and Victorian period scripting in her self-talk. So, she usually consents to being sexual with Jack, whether she wants to or not. It's just not worth the struggle and argument if she doesn't go along with his desire. This is usually an assumption on her behalf.

When they start interacting sexually, there is underlying tension between them. They aren't relaxed with each other. On a conscious level, Jack doesn't want to acknowledge this tension; he just wants to have sex. This is not to say that he is unaware that Sue has a hurry-up-and-get-it-over-with attitude, so he proceeds with a very goal-oriented style of touching, doing just enough so that it appears that Sue is ready to have intercourse. He focuses his touching primarily on her breasts and genitals, with very little foreplay. Once she seems ready, Jack gets on top in the missionary position. He continues to sense Sue's tension; even though she may be a good actress, the act eventually wears thin. As a result, Jack doesn't last long before ejaculating. He isn't able to relax and enjoy whatever sexual pleasure he is experiencing; all he can really do is relieve his sexual tension, just as he would if he were masturbating.

As for Sue, the experience provides little, if any, sexual pleasure. On occasions when she starts to get excited, he usually ejaculates before she can really get into the experience; so, after a while, she stops herself from becoming aroused to avoid the frustration. After he ejaculates, he rolls over and goes to sleep. She may get a pleasurable feeling being physically close to her husband for a period of time and give him a good night kiss. Sue feels relieved that she has satisfied Jack for the moment, but the next night the whole process begins again. It's as if he is a bottomless pit of sexual satisfaction. Each time she consents to this type of sexual experience with her husband, she is left feeling resentment and frustration, which continue to build over time. These unresolved emotions will continue to create an intimacy void between them.

This type of sexual interaction is an example of what I call meat-and-potatoes sex. Jack and Sue are engaging in "junk sex," from which they get as much real nourishment as they'd expect to get from eating burgers and fries at the local fast food restaurant every night. There may be nothing wrong with junk food or junk sex once in a while, but a steady diet of it is unhealthy and deadening to the palate. It also gets boring doing the same thing over and over. When you've gotten a quick fix at the fast-food restaurant, you're satisfied for the moment, but several hours later, you're hungry again. Doesn't this describe Jack's sexual experience? In a way, he is suffering from sexual malnutrition. He is always sexually starved because when he is sexual with Sue, it leaves him unfulfilled. This is the reason that he seems to have such a high sex drive. This could be said for a lot of men especially.

Continuing the metaphor, my advice to Jack and Sue would be to stop the junk food habit, save up their money, and choose an evening to go to the best restaurant in town. I would recommend a well-known French restaurant, for example. When I go to a restaurant like this with my wife, the dinner is the event for the night. It's not like I am grabbing a bite to eat, and then heading off to the show or concert. When you spend a lot of money going out for dinner, you're not going to gobble it up in 15 minutes. You're much more likely to savor every bite. First there is the salad, then the soup, then the main entrée, followed by dessert. Before you know it, a couple of hours have gone by. Sometimes, the dinner has gone on so long that your rear end is sore from sitting in one place.

You might ask how this metaphor relates to Jack and Sue's sexual relationship. If they were to take my advice, the following changes would take place: First, they would make love more slowly and leisurely. I'd say to Jack, "What's the hurry? Slow it all down. You should savor something so pleasurable." Make love just like the dinner experience I described previously. Second, they would spend more time touching—but without any goals except for the pleasure of the moment. Both would then begin to experience more pleasure.

As their sexual pleasure increases, Jack and Sue's whole relationship changes. Jack's seemingly insatiable sex drive suddenly seems to have been satisfied. If you've ever had a dinner experience I described earlier, you think or fantasize about eating this type of gourmet food all the time. In reality though, it would be too rich, and you would become obese. With this type of eating experience, an individual is not as likely to want to eat that type of food the next night because they are still satisfied and full from the previous night's eating experience.

This is what's happening to Jack, only on a sexual level. Because he now is experiencing a great deal of sustained sexual pleasure, he isn't so turned on the next night. Even though he might fantasize about having sex all the time, the reality is something different; he is feeling sexually satisfied. One positive consequence of Jack's increase of sexual pleasure in his love life with Sue is that his seemingly insatiable sex drive is satisfied, and his need for sex decreases. He stops pressuring Sue to be sexually involved every night. Sue's sexual interest increases with the increase of sexual pleasure. Now, she starts initiating sexual activity, since Jack no longer pressures her every night. Jack's more relaxed posture gives Sue a chance to come on to him for a change. Also, there is more motivation for Sue to initiate sex with Jack because he isn't in such a hurry as he was in the past. The tension between them is gone because Sue is interested in being sexual; Jack is now more relaxed, and as a result, doesn't ejaculate as fast when they have intercourse.

To summarize: As Jack and Sue develop their taste for "gourmet" sex, Jack lets go of his compulsive intensity where sex is concerned, and Sue's sexual interest starts to increase. Over time, their desires will begin to balance. When the level of sexual pleasure in a relationship increases, sexual satisfaction stays high—but not at a level that would reflect insatiable desire on the part of either or both partners. Extreme frequency of sexual activity is generally the result of one of the partners trying to play out their fantasies, or of the lack of real sexual quality or satisfaction in a relationship.

In the final analysis, questions of frequency generally give way to questions of quality. Quality in a sexual experience equates with the degree of sexual pleasure. If there is quality in our experiences when we do have sex, we don't usually keep score, nor do we compulsively come back again and again, night after night, attempting to satisfy a misguided appetite. The most satisfying sexual relationships aren't like ballgames, where the person scoring the most points wins. They're more like vacations, where goals are forgotten, and there is time to savor the varied delights of the senses that deepen intimacy and ease the small tensions of daily life.

Sex as a Measure of Emotional Intimacy

Another reason for problems with sexual frequency is the lack of emotional intimacy in the relationship. It is very difficult—if not impossible—for a couple to go from essentially being roommates outside their bedroom to going into their bedroom and becoming passionate, sexual lovers. This is especially true for women because they are conditioned with the belief that in order to interact sexually, they need to experience some type of emotional caring and regard from their partner. Men, on the other hand, don't get the same message that they have to be emotionally involved with a woman in order to be sexually involved. Yes, the double standard still exists.

Women tell their partners that they need to have some emotional communication before they can be sexually active. Men typically respond that they want to be sexually involved first, and then maybe they will communicate intimately. This is the classic standoff that interferes with sexual frequency.

This difference between men and women regarding sexual activity generally only applies when there has been an official commitment to the relationship. In the dating or courtship phase, there might be a great deal of sexual activity between the couple, even though there is a limited amount of emotional intimacy. This is a major contrast to the way it was before the mid-1960s. Today, women can be just as sexually active as their male counterparts. This often seems to change, though, once they get married because they need to feel the emotional intimacy within the marital context in order to be sexually active.

If partners in a couple are not close emotionally, they can cover up the fact by appearing to be good parents, friends, and social partners. From the outside—and perhaps even to themselves—they appear to be a happy couple. But the appearance is only superficial. One thing they can't cover up is what happens in the bedroom—which is usually very little. In their case, sexual frequency becomes the problem. It is easier for them to identify this obvious symptom as their problem than it is for them to talk about the cause, which is lack of emotional intimacy in their marriage.

Often, couples who feel they have a problem with frequency will try to increase their sexual desire. In the past, they might have rented adult videos from the local video store. With the advent of the Internet and the demise of the video store, access to explicit adult content has become even easier than ever.

The couple's intent is that by watching other people in very explicit sexual activity, they will become aroused themselves, so that then they will want to make love. Now, I have nothing against watching adult films or video clips, but I don't believe any couple should rely on this method to provide greater sexual activity between them. I don't like it when a couple relies on any one variable to create sexual desire. It's too rigid and will eventually lose its stimulating factor. Most likely, they aren't addressing the real underlying psychological issue and are just treating the symptom; i.e., lack of sexual desire, superficially.

Sometimes, people try to increase their sexual frequency and desire by using drugs and alcohol. Drugs like marijuana, cocaine, and ecstasy particularly can be used to temporarily remove blocks to emotional closeness, so that the couple can then be physically close. Alcohol works the same way, unless you drink too much—then you don't feel anything sexually and just fall asleep. Again, if using chemicals is the only way that a couple can be sexually close, then the actual problem isn't being addressed. This is most likely the lack of emotional intimacy between the couple, perhaps stemming from some other unresolved personal issues from the past.

Women's Headaches or Men's Headaches?

Generally, when the subject of sexual frequency comes up for discussion, most people assume that it is the woman who isn't interested in sex. After all, she is always the one depicted in the popular media as having a headache and is the brunt of many a comedian's joke. In my clinical experience, however, this is not necessarily the case. In fact, it seems that I see many more men who lack sexual interest, usually men aged 45 and up. Women seldom tell me that they are not interested in sex, unless they are in that "wonderful period" of their life called menopause. But they often say that in order to have physical intimacy, they first need to have some type of an intimate emotional connection with their husband. Without that psychological connection, they are turned off to being sexually involved.

Males in their forties and beyond often keep looking for that sexual urge or desire to motivate them to be involved sexually. Without that sexual urge, they get distracted by other nonerotic activities, such as golf, television, and, of course, their work. The sexual urge is driven by the sexual hormone testosterone. By the time a male reaches his late forties, the degree of testosterone he produces has decreased since he was in his twenties and thirties. Besides that biological fact, a man's lifestyle may not help him regarding testosterone production. High levels of anxiety and the commitment he has to his work inhibit the hormone's production. The repression of anger and its associated depression also play a role in reducing his testosterone levels. The bottom line is that the sexual urge isn't there like it used to be when he was younger. If the requirement for his sexual initiation or participation is experiencing the sexual urge before he has sex, then the frequency will greatly be reduced.

Anger and Sexual Desire

The most common inhibitors of sexual desire are the emotions of anger, hurt, and resentment. It isn't the emotions themselves that cause the sexual inhibition, but how they are dealt with inside the relationship. The most common method of expressing these emotions for couples is to repress them and block their verbal communication. As a result of this lack of direct effective verbal communication, these resentments and anger become psychologically buried over time, and a buildup occurs.

The basic fact is that it's very difficult—if not impossible—to be sexually turned on, romantic, and affectionate with a partner when you are holding back anger, hurt, and resentment toward them. It doesn't matter if these emotions are related to something that happened five years ago, yesterday, or ten minutes ago. It doesn't matter how little or how big the anger is; if its expression and resolution are blocked, sexual activity won't be happening. Nobody is can enjoy intimacy and sexual closeness until the anger has been dealt with in a satisfactory manner.

Unfortunately, many people are uncomfortable expressing or receiving anger, so rather than dealing with it, they ignore or repress it. Many people heard this parental message when they were growing up: "If you don't have anything nice to say, then don't say anything at all." This message isn't directed specifically to anger, but for most people in Western culture, anger and resentment are viewed as negative emotions. So, if this is what you feel emotionally, then society discourages you from expressing it. If my grandmother were alive, I would tell her that this was a very dysfunctional concept, at least within the context of an intimate relationship. It might make sense at Thanksgiving or Christmas with relatives I only see once a year and where there is no intention of developing an intimate relationship. Yes, at the holidays we can have a very nice time and a nice dinner and everyone can be nice to each other, but this doesn't work with a lover. Holding back anger and hurt only blocks the occurrence of emotional and sexual intimacy.

Another concept I've heard about in the last few years is an attitude that seems to be reinforced by the self-help book, *Don't Sweat the Small Stuff*, by Richard Carlson.(3) His book is full of good cognitive concepts, but I think many people just took the title as reinforcement for an attitude that is problematic as it relates to the management of resentments. Many people say to themselves or to their lover that their resentment about something is petty, trivial, or stupid, or that they are just overreacting. Basically, they are saying don't sweat the small resentments, and repress the emotions. The problem is that all the small resentments in a relationship tend to collect and build over time. It's as if the person is not conscious of these resentments as they walk around in their daily life, but every once in a while, things erupt emotionally over what seems like a small incident. That small incident detonates the big bomb of resentment and anger that is under the psychological surface, waiting for something to set it off. It is these small resentments that can lead to the demise of the intimacy and sexual desire within a committed relationship.

One aspect of a relationship where the repression of resentments and anger take their toll is when it comes to the amount of physical affection expressed between the couple. When a couple is in the early courtship phase and when they are newly married, there is a great deal of physical affection between them. They are always touching each other, both privately and in public. Sometimes, they make others around them uncomfortable with all their displays of affection.

Once a couple is married and has spent a couple of years together, it's common for the degree of expression of physical affection to decrease. This is such a common occurrence that married couples just rationalize this change with "That's just the way it is when you get married."

I don't believe that's the way it has to be. I see the lack of affection as a direct result of the way couples deal with resentments between them that occur from just living together day after day. Generally, these resentments are small, and therefore they get repressed. The resentment sometimes is large, but if it gets repressed, that same result occurs: little affection.

When couples first get together, there is not a large amount of resentment built up between them, and when they are together, they just want to touch each other because it feels so good. So, if they start touching each other in the kitchen and the pleasure builds, sexual activity becomes a major possibility. On the contrary, when they have been together for an extended period of time, the resentments have been collected and psychologically repressed between them. Instead of feeling pleasure when her husband touches her, a wife feels irritated by his touch and wants him to leave her alone. She might say something like, "Do you have to touch me? You know I am busy making dinner. Stop bothering me with all this affection now." People don't like to be touched when they are resentful or angry. Instead, they want physical space—not closeness or intimacy—until their resentment and anger have been resolved.

My Attitude Shift Regarding Anger Within an Intimate Relationship

One of the first things I told my lovers when things between us were getting serious was "If I do anything that you resent, whether it's tiny or huge, I want you to tell me as soon as possible. I won't get upset at you if I can help it." They would sometimes respond: "Are you crazy? You want me to tell you when you piss me off? Won't you think I'm just being bitchy? Are you a masochist?" "Absolutely not; I just don't want you to turn off to me sexually. If you hold back your resentments and anger, I know you will shut down your sexual desire and responsiveness when you are with me sexually." Eventually, they would trust my request with "Okay, I know you like sex, so I will take the risk and tell you when I am resentful or angry."

Before I trained as a sex therapist, my attitude regarding the expression of anger in a relationship was quite different. This attitude is quite common with many men I deal with in therapy and with male college students. My attitude was basically: "Don't bother me with your anger and resentments. They are petty and irrational. Leave me alone. I don't want to hear your nagging about my behavior." This attitude began with my mother and was probably a coping mechanism. I can remember yelling at her to leave me alone and stop telling me to turn my stereo volume down.

I could blow off my mother's anger and resentment and tell her I didn't want to hear it without any severe consequences. Intimacy with my mother was not an issue. We were in a major power struggle, with her holding most of the cards because I was still dependent on her for emotional and financial security. If I took the same attitude about resentment and anger I had with my mother and applied it to a marital relationship, the emotional and sexual intimacy would have died over time. So what works in one psychological context may not work in another.

Call Your Wife or Girlfriend a Bitch and Say Good-Bye to Your Love Life

Often in a relationship, when a woman expresses her anger, her partner will judge her as being a bitch for being angry. It's not acceptable in our culture for women to express anger, no matter how they communicate the emotion. When they do express anger, they take a big psychological risk because most likely they will be judged and called a bitch.

When a male partner calls his lover a bitch, he is basically telling her that she can't express anger. He wants her to just smile and be happy. Good luck. What he doesn't realize is that when his lover shuts down her anger because she doesn't want to be called a bitch, she won't want to express her anger and resentments again. When her anger and resentments become repressed, she will, in turn, shut down her sexual desire within their relationship; they will both miss out on having a passionate, highly responsive sex life.

The repression of resentments and anger can take their toll in the dating world as well. I am told often in therapy, "You know, Dan, my sexual relationships start off being so exciting, but after a month or so they just become humdrum; I don't understand why." My response is that after a couple spends some time together, they start to irritate each other with specific behaviors. It's only natural for this to happen. Since they have just started dating, they usually don't want to express any resentments.

They are overwhelmed by the wonderful infatuation they are experiencing and don't want to destroy the joy and pleasure they are feeling by expressing their resentments, so instead they repress. After a month or so, this blocking process begins to take its toll on the couple's sexual responsiveness, both in and out of bed.

Most single people who find themselves in this situation just write it off to boredom with the relationship. They decide it is time to move on to another person. They never seem to realize why the pattern of excitement followed by boredom keeps repeating itself. When this happens to a married couple, they can't so easily move on to another relationship, so they find other activities to occupy their interest. This shift in their attention will only last so long until their relationship implodes and dissolves—unless they get help with how to express their resentments and open up the channels of passion again.

Power Struggles and the Lack of Sexual Desire

The most common source of anger in a long-term relationship is a power struggle between the partners. Whatever the couple is struggling over—such as money, sex, or how they might discipline their children—the struggle for power and control affects their level of intimacy. Intimacy, either emotional or physical, can't really develop when power and control are the driving forces between a couple.

When the battle for power and control occurs, regardless of what the contention is, the couple become adversaries. As Helen Singer Kaplan states, "Regardless of origin of anger, it is not possible for most persons to feel sexual desire for the enemy. Repressed anger and love act as mutual inhabitants."(4) Partners involved in a power struggle give up their need to be close and intimate because they don't really want the intimacy; they would rather win the battle. But even if they win the battle, they lose the relationship, at least in terms of being lovers.

As we have seen, quality sex requires vulnerability. If partners are competing for control, the last thing they want to do is be vulnerable, lower their defenses, and abandon themselves to sexual pleasure. Instead, it is safer to block their feelings of sexual desire and protect themselves psychologically from their partner.

Some couples report to me that after they get angry with each other, being critical and yelling and calling each other names, they start to have sexual feelings toward each other. Often, these feelings lead to a very intense sexual experience. Some people call this makeup sex because it usually occurs after a couple has made up after an argument or fight.

This type of sexual experience occurs for several reasons. One is that the couple has probably released repressed anger during their argument; it was getting in the way of their sexual desire. That's why couples who do a great deal of talking about their resentments tend to have greater sexual frequency in their marriage than couples who never fight.

I don't want to suggest that in order to have a high frequency of sexual activity in a marriage, you should yell and scream at each other. On the contrary, it is good to express your resentments and anger with your partner, but do so in a constructive manner, preferably using "I" messages as opposed to "you" messages. This style of communication is discussed in further detail in my book, *Creating the Intimate Connection: The Basics of Emotional Intimacy.*(5)

While yelling and screaming may work for the moment, releasing anger so that sexual desire may come to the surface will bury desire in the long run. This is because when a couple communicates in such a coarse, ineffective way, they usually hurt each other in the process. Eventually, this hurt will accumulate into emotional scar tissue, which blocks sexual desire.

Sometimes, when partners have expressed their anger aggressively, they want to be close because of fear. They are each afraid that, having yelled or called the other names, they have hurt their lover (and, of course, they have), and therefore the lover might leave or abandon them. As a way to compensate for this fear, they reach out and become sexually close. What better way to assuage these fears of abandonment than by having sexual intercourse? This pattern only happens if both partners experience the fear of abandonment. It may work for a while, but eventually the pattern will break down, because you can only hurt someone for so long before that person will stop wanting to be close. The breakdown will occur more rapidly as a person's self-esteem increases and, as a result, the fear of being abandoned or living alone decreases.

Relationship Issues That Block Sexual Frequency

Emotional intimacy is the prerequisite for sexual frequency. When it is absent, sexual frequency drops off. Let's look briefly at other relationship issues that also affect a couple's sexual frequency.

The first issue is that of trust. There has to be a fundamental trust between partners for them to have a quality sexual relationship over a period of time. They have to trust that their partner/lover is not out to hurt them in any way—that their partner is committed to the relationship, meaning that their partner isn't contemplating leaving soon, and is not sexually or emotionally involved with someone else—and that their partner will be there to give emotional support if they make themselves vulnerable and communicate their emotions. At the core of the matter is the trust that one is being accepted and that the atmosphere is free of judgment.

Trust has to do not only with trusting your partner, but with trusting yourself as well. You must be able to trust yourself to maintain your own sense of identity before you can become emotionally intimate with a lover. Otherwise, you will tend to cave in or sell out on your needs or wants because you are afraid that you won't be loved if you create a conflict. Also, you must have trust or confidence in yourself that once you do become emotionally vulnerable, if the relationship becomes detrimental to your mental health, you will be able to terminate the relationship.

Without trust in all its forms, emotional vulnerability cannot flourish. Without vulnerability, sexual quality is usually poor, and as a consequence, sexual frequency drops off.

Another source of resentment that blocks sexual desire is a longing for romance—a desire for the close, loving attention that usually comes in the early stages of dating. Alan and Donna Brauer write: "When women are sexually frustrated and miss the positive romantic attention they feel they need, we've found they become withdrawn, depressed, or angry. In a word, irritable. This reaction, which is often unconscious, may lead them to start arguments over issues that are seemingly unrelated. That sounds irrational, but it operates by the logic of frustration: at least their arguing makes their partners pay attention, and better angry attention than none at all."(6)

Regular romantic input and intimacy can go a long way toward reducing the level of frustration and resentment in the relationship. This needs to be a part of daily living—not just an awkward flourish on special occasions or an obligatory gesture just before bed.

In the final analysis, questions of frequency generally give way to questions of quality. If there is quality in our experiences when we do have sex, we don't usually keep score, nor do we compulsively come back again and again, night after night, attempting to satisfy a misguided appetite. The most satisfying sexual relationships aren't like ballgames, where the person scoring the most points wins. They are more like vacations, where goals are forgotten and there is time to savor the varied delights of the senses that deepen intimacy and erase the petty tensions of daily life.

Works Cited

1. http://www.amazines.com/view_author.cfm?authorid=841410&Author=David&20Atkins
2. http://www.amazines.com/view_author.cfm?authorid=841410&Author=David&20Atkins
3. Carlson, Richard. *Don't Sweat the Small Stuff.* New York: Hyperion, 1997.
4. Singer Kaplan, Helen, MD, PhD. *The New Sex Therapy.* New York: Taylor and Francis Group, 1974.

5. Beaver, Daniel. *Creating the Intimate Connection: The Basics of Emotional Intimacy.* San Diego: Cognella, 2011.
6. Brauer, Alan, & Brauer, Donna. *ESO: How You and Your Lover Can Give Each Other Hours of Extended Sexual Orgasms.* New York: Wellness Central, Hachette Book Group, 2001.

10

Sexual Dysfunctions

Causes and Treatment for Men

This chapter and the next deal with sexual dysfunctions. My purpose is to familiarize you with the common sexual problems that we all may encounter in our lives. I also want to provide some understanding of the causes of these dysfunctions and some of the ways they can be treated. Since it is difficult to treat our own sexual problems without the help of a trained professional, I don't intend this information to be employed in self-treatment. Rather, my purpose is to help readers recognize certain dysfunctions and know there are successful treatments available. Sexual problems don't get better with time; they only worsen if not treated.

Many sexual dysfunctions, particularly those of males, could be prevented if men had a better understanding of their own sexuality. As Dr. Bernie Zilbergeld states in his book, *Male Sexuality*, "The models of sex and masculinity that were and are presented to us are deficient in a great many ways, harmful to both us and our partners, and the main cause of our sexual dissatisfaction and problems. These models have little to do with what is possible or satisfying for human beings."(1) I would like to add that the same things are true for most women.

Sexual dysfunction is a very broad subject, not one that could be completely covered in a book of this kind. For this reason, I have chosen to explore only the more common issues. Sex therapists and others wishing to have more extensive clinical information will, I'm afraid, have to go elsewhere for that. My intention here is to provide a survey of common dysfunctions and their available treatment, not to offer a comprehensive clinical picture.

In the past, many mental health professionals viewed all sexual dysfunctions as symptomatic of deep-seated psychological problems. The treatment of these problems required intensive, long-term psychotherapy that delved into a patient's childhood to uncover the roots of the problem. The results of this therapeutic process were questionable at best. The approach was based on the traditional Freudian psychoanalytic theories that sexual problems were manifested in adult life because the individual was fixated in a certain stage of development during childhood. The cure was based on the discovery of when this fixation occurred. It could take years to reach a conclusion, and the results of this therapeutic approach were debatable.

The psychoanalytic approach to treating sexual dysfunctions for both men and women was the only way the medical community treated sexual problems for the first half of the 20th century. Then, a new approach emerged at the Department of Obstetrics and Gynecology at Washington University in St. Louis, Missouri. This approach was developed by a research team composed of William H. Masters and Virginia E. Johnson, who pioneered research into the nature of human sexual response and the diagnosis and treatment of sexual disorders and dysfunctions from 1957 until the 1990s.

Masters and Johnson developed what we now call sex therapy and radically altered the approach to treating sexual dysfunctions. They advocated a treatment approach that dealt with the patient's sexual life in the present, focusing on changing the patient's sexual behavior by prescribing exercises for couples to do outside the therapist's office. Their therapy lasted two weeks and often generated immediate results. Much of what I will be describing in this chapter is drawn from my professional training that came from Masters and Johnson.

Like many other sex therapists, I have taken the sex therapy program developed by Masters and Johnson and adapted it to my own style and clinical practice. For instance, I usually see a couple once a week while they are participating in their normal lifestyle of work and raising a family. Masters and Johnson saw a couple every day for two weeks and the patients stayed in a local hotel near their clinic. Typically, they would have a team of male and female co-therapists. I usually work by myself for practical reasons such as affordability of therapy and the couple's availability.

Men's Common Sexual Problems: Symptoms and Solutions

Erectile Dysfunction

When Masters and Johnson did their research and published their second book, *Human Sexual Inadequacy*,(2) the term erectile dysfunction wasn't used, but instead they used the term impotence. Generally, this sexual dysfunction is characterized by the inability to develop or maintain an erection of the penis during sexual performance. The incidence of this dysfunction increases in men as they age, especially after the age of 60.

Erectile dysfunction, or ED, is probably the most frustrating and humiliating sexual dysfunction a man can experience. The term impotence that was used in the past gives some clue as to the psychological impact on the person experiencing this difficulty.

The word impotence has such a negative psychological connotation that further aggravates the problem. When a male is unable to achieve or maintain an erection, he feels worthless as a man, and his self-esteem takes a major hit. To say that a man is impotent is to suggest powerlessness, a label that carries over into his feelings about his abilities in other areas of his life. For this reason, I like the change of labels to erectile dysfunction that is currently being used.

When a man isn't able to achieve or maintain an erection, he usually becomes upset and angry about his ability to perform. He may internalize this anger, which then creates feelings of depression. When someone is depressed, it suppresses their testosterone production. When this occurs in men, their ability to achieve an erection is negatively affected. It all becomes a vicious cycle of erectile dysfunction.

Erectile problems can occur in either of two ways. One is acute, or situational, erectile inadequacy, in which the man who has had past success in attaining and maintaining erections is suddenly unable to do so. The second form of erectile inadequacy is chronic, in which the man has had a long history of inability to attain and maintain erections. In the past, the chronic type was more difficult to correct. In some cases, this is still true, but with the advent of ED medications, cure rates have increased.

The physiological aspect of ED is an impairment of the erectile reflex. The vascular reflex mechanism fails to pump a sufficient amount of blood into the body of the penis to fill and render the penis erect. This impairment usually occurs at the point when the male experiences a great deal of emotional anxiety about his sexual performance. The reaction can happen any time during the sexual response cycle.

At least half the male population experiences erection difficulties at one time or another. In the first large-scale study to assess age and erectile function, researchers from the Harvard School of Public Health found that ED is common among older men and increases with age. They also found that men who were physically active and stayed lean had a lower prevalence of ED. The findings appear in the August 5, 2003, issue of the *Annals of Internal Medicine*.(3)

In the past, when men had difficulties with erections, they were very reluctant to talk about it with their friends or spouses. They would hide the fact that they were having problems. There was so much shame and embarrassment surrounding this sexual dysfunction that they would just deny its existence by not being involved in any sexual activity to avoid the embarrassment and the sense of inadequacy. Their sex lives typically ended with the diagnosis of ED. With the advent of sex therapy in the mid-1970s, some men began seeking treatment for the problem, but the vast majority just hid their difficulty. With the discovery of ED medications, males with erectile difficulties came out of hiding about their struggle and began to address the problem with their medical doctors.

Common Psychological Reactions to ED

The psychological impact of ED is potentially tremendous. The degree of impact has a lot to do with how knowledgeable the man is about his own sexuality, and particularly how aware he is of his own conditions for being sexually functional. In other words, the more knowledge he has, the better he will be able to accept and understand his problem. Only a few men who came to me for help started out with this kind of knowledge and understanding.

When a man cannot get or maintain an erection, he usually feels inadequate as a man, lover, or husband. He questions his own masculinity and self-esteem. So it is not much of an overstatement to say that, for a man, everything in the world depends on the performance of his penis. As Zilbergeld states in *Male Sexuality*, "The erection is considered by almost all men as the star performer in the drama of sex, and we all know what happens to a show when the star performer doesn't make an appearance. The whole show is cancelled or, to be a bit more accurate, the planned performance gives way to an impromptu tragedy, replete with wailing and self-blaming, usually ending with everyone feeling miserable."(4)

When a man has problems maintaining an erection, he becomes extremely self-critical. The internal psychological critical parent voice starts blaring in his ear. The internal dialogue might go something like this: "What's the matter with you? Why don't you work, damn it? You're just over the hill! She is going to leave you if don't get it up, you jerk!"

When a man talks to his penis in this manner, the penis just shuts down and doesn't want to participate in being sexual. This only infuriates the man further, and it becomes a vicious cycle. The consequence of this self-attack is a confusing combination of resentment, feelings of inadequacy, and anxiety, followed by depression and a sense of hopelessness. The part of the man that is afraid he won't be able to sustain an erection is like a frightened child. Another part is demanding and worried about his pride and ego. This part doesn't allow for imperfection and mistakes. I liken this part to a critical parent.

When a child is afraid to do something, the last thing a parent should do is yell at him. All this does is traumatize the child even more. But this is exactly how the internal critical parent behaves for a man who is having erection difficulties. It yells at the part of him that is a frightened child. The critical parent may so intimidate the inner child that he doesn't want to be sexually involved at all, for fear of failure and further punishment.

Depression, Testosterone, and ED

One common symptom of a male's insecurity about his ability to achieve erections is a secondary depression. As a result of all his self-loathing, he develops a great deal of repressed anger. This, in turn, translates into psychological depression, whose physiological effects create a vicious circle.

The presence of testosterone in the bloodstream activates the brain to cause erotic desire and motivation. At the same time, testosterone provides the chemical environment necessary for sperm production, ejaculation, and erections. Of course, testosterone is not the sole determinant for these phenomena—psychological and social influences also play their parts—but it does have an important function to perform.

A male's psychological state influences his testosterone level, which fluctuates considerably in response to psychic and sexual stimulation. When a male is in a state of depression, defeat, humiliation, or in high-anxiety situations, the secretion of testosterone drops off. As we have just seen, a man who is having difficulty with erections is likely to have precisely these feelings. His psychological state sets off a psychological reaction, which reinforces the very problem that is making him depressed and anxious. The greater his reaction, the worse the problem becomes.

The Partner's Role

Erectile dysfunction also has a psychological impact on the man's partner. Again, the degree of impact is related to his partner's level of sexual experience and to her confidence in her own sexuality.

Many women will be sympathetic and will try to downplay the situation. Of course, her message may fall upon deaf ears because her partner is so absorbed in self-loathing.

If a man's partner is not confident in her own sexuality, his inability to maintain erections may threaten her. She will begin to feel responsible and start questioning herself. "Is this because of the way I look? He doesn't think I'm sexy anymore. Maybe he is involved with somebody else." These doubts take their emotional toll on her by creating fear and anxiety, which may make it difficult for her to be sexually involved.

Some women will try to rescue the man from his sexual performance problem. They may see themselves as a sexual Florence Nightingale, committed to curing the man from his affliction of ED. They may try all sorts of techniques to arouse their partner to get an erection. His problem becomes her responsibility, and her ego gets involved along with his.

Like those who play the rescuer/codependent role in other personal relationships, the woman eventually tires of trying to fix the victim's problem; she becomes frustrated and angry over the lack of results. At first, she is very motivated and reassuring, but as one effort after another fails, she becomes agitated and critical of her partner. This criticism quickly drives him further into self-loathing.

Some women try to rescue their partners from ED in a different way. Instead of taking a direct approach and taking responsibility for his problem, a woman might try to protect him from his problem by not confronting the situation at all. She might treat the man like a child who is too fragile to deal with the real world. She withholds the consequences of the problem and thus prevents him from having to face the situation and seeking psychological help to resolve his issue. This approach is called enabling, where an individual reinforces behavior that they don't like in their partner by not giving them consequences.

This rescuing pattern seems to work for a while, in that there is no confrontation or conflict. On the surface, the relationship seems stable. But meanwhile, there is no sex for either partner. Over time, this unmet need creates much hurt and anger for the woman and a sense of depression for her partner. If sex is at all important to her, this resentment will build, and she will eventually explode. When this happens, her male partner will probably react by feeling overwhelmed and defensive and will retreat into a deeper depression and wall off to her even more.

The message in all this is that any form of codependent behavior by the partner is invariably nonproductive. No matter what a woman partner does or says, it is the man's problem, and he has to take responsibility for his own sexuality and finding a solution. He will feel a great amount of pressure no matter what she does because of his own expectations of himself.

When I say it is his problem, I don't want to imply that the female partner is unaffected. It is just that her problem is a different one. Her problem is the lack of sexual frequency due to his avoidance of sexual activity. This is a problem that she can do something about. Getting angry with her partner does little to correct it. What she needs to do is direct her anger at the situation she finds herself in. She can change her situation with or without her partner's help.

The woman's best option would be to immediately confront her partner with her feelings about their relationship. A good approach is to suggest that they get into some sort of therapy—preferably sex therapy—so that their problems can be remedied before they become worse. She could also suggest that he seek medical advice to see whether he has any medical issues contributing to the problem. If he won't participate in any type of psychological therapy or medical help, then she needs to explain to him the consequences to their relationship if the problem goes unresolved.

Confronting the Psychological Causes of Erectile Insecurity

The psychological cause at the onset of erection difficulties is often that the man's conditions for sexual functioning are not being met. When his penis does not want to become erect, it is, in a sense, saying something to its owner, perhaps that it is not comfortable with the conditions of intimacy with his female partner. The male may not be ready to listen to what his penis is saying because he thinks the conditions shouldn't matter; if there is a sexual opportunity for intercourse, then his penis should just work on demand.

The conditions required for adequate sexual functioning vary from person to person, but here are some common ones that I have dealt with in my work.

A man must feel emotionally comfortable with the woman he is sexually involved with if he is to function properly on a sexual level. He may have built-up resentments that he hasn't communicated to his partner that make it difficult for him to become aroused enough to maintain an erection. The man also needs to be able to trust the emotional commitment of his partner. This is a problem for many single men who are trying to be sexually involved with women who are also seeing other men. This can also be an issue when a man fears that his wife may be involved with another man.

Often, when a married man is having a sexual affair, he has difficulties with erections. I ask him, "Are you emotionally comfortable in this relationship?" and he answers, "Sure, she is great looking and we can talk about all kinds of things."

The rest of the dialogue will usually go something like this:

"Yes, but are you emotionally comfortable?"

"What's that got to do with getting a hard-on? You should see what a great body she has! I just don't know what my problem is."

"How do you feel when you are with her and not with your wife?"

"Well, at first it's exciting to be with her, but after a while I start to feel guilty and become somewhat anxious about my wife finding out about this other relationship and kicking me out of the house."

So, I persist in questioning, and finally, the patient starts to really express his emotions. On the surface, things appear to be okay, but underneath he is feeling guilty and anxious. These feelings are getting in the way of his ability to function adequately sexually.

I tell men in this situation that they are responding normally to an uncomfortable sexual situation. Hearing this can be comforting to some men because they feel so inadequate and abnormal. For others, it can be hard to hear because they think they should be able to function adequately under whatever psychological conditions that exist within the relationship.

This misconception that many men hold to, which says that they should be able to have sex at any time and any place with anyone, sets them up for sexual problems. They think that having conditions is for women, not men. This may have been true when a man was 18 or 20 and his biological drives were going full blast and overruling his emotional conditions. But as he moves into his thirties, forties, and beyond, his sexuality is influenced more and more by his emotional environment. The more a man fights this fact, the greater the odds that he will experience sexual difficulties.

The fact remains that when emotional conditions aren't met, many men have difficulty with erections. As natural as this sounds, many men don't want to believe it. Then, when the causes of the problem aren't addressed and the erectile difficulties continue, other factors come into play, making matters worse. In Chapter Eleven, I discuss these other factors in greater detail.

There are some men who have psychological issues with their fear of commitment to a relationship and fear of emotional intimacy with their partner that can cause them erectile difficulties. Men with these issues perform better with women when there is no chance of emotional intimacy or concerns about commitment, such as a one-night stand or sex with a prostitute.

Physical Causes of Erectile Dysfunctions

When I treat men for ED, my first task is to rule out any medical conditions involved that might be contributing to their sexual problem. Of all the male sexual dysfunctions, ED may have the most physical contributors involved.

It's common for men to think right away that their erection problem is related to something physical because they don't want to admit that the problem could be psychological. Most of the time the sexual problem of ED has a psychological basis, but I want to make sure that nothing medical is involved before I move ahead with psychological therapy.

One physical issue to check for is whether the individual is under emotional stress in his daily life. Stress at work or stress in his home can carry over into his bedroom, having a negative impact on his sexual performance.

When an individual says they are experiencing stress in their life, what they are really saying is that they are experiencing the emotion of anxiety. When a male is anxious, it's hard for him to relax and enjoy the pleasure of the moment. He won't be able to experience sexual pleasure and will have difficulties with erections. Then he will have anxiety about his inability to perform, and that will, in turn, make the sexual problem worse. And the vicious cycle begins.

Another condition that comes from being stressed out and experiencing a great deal of anxiety is fatigue. If a male is exhausted, this condition doesn't lend itself to achieving and maintaining an erection because it's pretty hard to enjoy any activity if you are ready to fall asleep at any moment.

Early undiagnosed diabetes can also impact a male's ability to have successful erections. "It is been estimated that about 35%–75% of men with diabetes will experience at least some degree of erectile dysfunction during their lifetime. The causes of erectile dysfunction in men with diabetes are complex and involve impairments in nerve, blood vessel, and muscle function.

"To get an erection, men need healthy blood vessels, nerves, male hormones, and a desire to be sexually stimulated. Diabetes can damage the blood vessels and nerves that control erection. Therefore, even if you have normal amounts of male hormones and you have the desire to have sex, you still may not be able to achieve a firm erection."(5)

The most common physical problem that men want to believe is that the cause of their erectile difficulties is a low level of testosterone in their blood supply. This used to be the medical belief as well, but there might be other issues involved other than the lack of testosterone.

"Testosterone is an important sex hormone, but there is no strong correlation between low testosterone levels and erectile dysfunction," explains Dr. J. Francois Eid, an American urologist. "A man's testosterone level affects his sexual desire, but it does not impact his ability to have an erection." Many studies shown that testosterone replacement has failed to benefit erectile function in men with normal or borderline low testosterone. Left untreated, erectile dysfunction can create a negative cycle whereby reduced incidence of erections leads to reduced sexual desire, which can be misinterpreted as low testosterone."(6)

Another common cause of erectile difficulties can be a male's use of alcohol and high blood pressure medications. Steady drinking can inhibit both erection and orgasm. It does so by affecting the production of nitrite oxide molecules, which, in turn, makes it difficult for the tissue of the corpus cavernosa to relax enough to allow blood to flow in the penis. If drinking continues over time and alcoholism develops, there is even more damage. The peripheral nervous system is often injured permanently, affecting the ability to have an erection.(7)

The problem with excessive alcohol consumption is that alcohol dilates the blood vessels in general, but specifically the penis. Dilation—as opposed to constriction—means that the blood vessels expand so much that the blood can't trap in the penis to render it erect. "During a typical erection, blood flows to the penis where more of it stays in than is released. Alcohol works to dilate blood vessels in the body, including in the penis. As a result, blood vessels in the penis stay open, blood flows out and the penis does not become rigid or achieves some degree of hardness but has difficulty staying firm."(8)

Researchers find that too much alcohol affects both your brain and your penis. In one University of Washington study, sober men were able to achieve an erection more quickly than intoxicated men—and some men are unable to have an erection *at all* after drinking. That's because pre-sex boozing decreases blood flow to your penis, reduces the intensity of your orgasm, and can dampen your level of excitement (in other words, even if you are able to have sex, it may not be nearly as pleasurable as it would be without the excess alcohol).(9)

One mistaken belief is that alcohol is a stimulant and can increase one's sexual performance. In fact, alcohol is a central nervous system depressant and dampens sexual arousal. It also numbs the nerve endings in the penis, leading to a decrease in both the intensity and pleasure in orgasm. Framed another way, your penis will pass out before you do.(10)

The most common medical cause of ED is reduced blood flow to the penis due to chronic conditions such as high blood pressure, high cholesterol, and hardening of the arteries. Since being able to achieve an erection is a vasocongestion event, a male's circulatory system needs to be in good shape in order to enjoy the experience.

The Typical Psychological Origin of Erection Difficulties

As with other sexual dysfunctions, a self-perpetuating loop or vicious circle is created. The following is a scenario typical of many men who have come to me with erection difficulties.

Jack and Sue are in their early thirties and have been married for about eight years. They have two small children, and both parents work outside of the home. After working hard all week, they decide to get a babysitter and go out to a friend's house for a party on Friday night.

As they are getting ready for the party, Jack is already feeling tired, but says to himself, "What the hell, we hired the babysitter, maybe I'll get a second wind."

While at the party, Jack and Sue have a great time, since it has been a while since they have been out alone together. Sue is a little concerned about how much Jack is drinking, though. They dance together and enjoy themselves, but by midnight, they have to leave to take the babysitter home.

By the time Jack gets back, Sue is waiting for him in bed with one of her sexy new negligees. She is feeling very amorous toward Jack after having such a good time together. Meanwhile, Jack is tired from the long day, plus the dancing, and is feeling the effects of several drinks. He knows that Sue wants to make love, but he is not feeling very energetic. He also knows that Sue doesn't initiate sexual activity very often, and he hates to turn her down. Also, he has always believed that he should always be ready to "get it on," regardless of when or where.

Jack gets into bed with Sue, and they start having fun sexually. But when they start to have intercourse, Jack loses his erection, and he and Sue stop being sexual with each other.

Sue says, "Don't worry about it, Jack. It's no big deal. You're just tired and probably had too much to drink. Let's just go to sleep." Jack feels embarrassed and sexually inadequate because this is the first time this has ever happened. He just wants to hide in a shell, so he rolls over and simply says good night.

The next day, the events of Friday night keep plaguing him. He can't wait for Saturday night to come because he wants to redeem himself and his sexual ego. He has been thinking about being sexual with Sue all day while he's been out on the soccer field with his kids. The level of anticipatory anxiety he is creating is very high. When it is finally time, he has been thinking about this moment all day.

When he gets in bed, he immediately starts pursuing Sue sexually. But while he is touching, kissing, and caressing her, his mind is focused not on the pleasure that he is receiving in the moment while he is touching her. Instead, he is paying attention to his penis—watching it, waiting for it to become erect so that he can have intercourse with Sue and make up for the sense of failure and inadequacy as a lover he still feels from the night before. It is as if his penis is on a stage with a big spotlight on it.

Jack's level of anxiety is enormous at this point. He has been thinking about getting an erection all day, and by the time he gets to the point of intercourse, his penis is under such an intense psychological spotlight that it simply shrinks off stage with stage fright. Jack is surprised and disappointed. He doesn't know what is wrong.

As time goes on, Jack keeps trying and trying to get an erection or to maintain one, to the point where he just can't take the humiliation and sense of inadequacy. He begins to avoid sex with Sue, making up excuses or claiming fatigue, when they both know what the real reason is. Neither of them knows what to do about the situation. They hope that with time the problem will go away, but it doesn't. It only gets worse with time.

The pattern I have just described is a common one. It can be avoided and corrected by the man, simply by gaining a more realistic understanding of his own sexuality. If his expectations of his penis were more in line with reality and less with the fantasy model of male sexuality perpetuated by North American culture, the problem would be avoided, or could be easily solved.

The erectile dysfunction pattern presented is another form of the classic goal-orientation loop. The goal is to achieve and maintain an erection. The more Jack works at trying to achieve his goal, the more anxiety he creates for himself. The more anxiety he experiences, the less pleasure he enjoys, and without the pleasure, he isn't able to obtain an erection, no matter how hard he tries. His goal-oriented approach keeps him from enjoying lovemaking because he is focused on his erection problem, rather than the pleasure of the moment. Jack is like a driver trying to free his car from a sand trap. The more the wheels spin to get out, the deeper the car sinks into the sand.

Jack must learn that he has psychological conditions that need to be met in order for him to function sexually. One of the biggest conditions is that he be able to relax and be free of sexual anxiety. He needs to learn that he can't just perform sexually any place, any time, with anybody. Just because he has the opportunity for intercourse doesn't mean he can perform. He is not a sex machine. He has thoughts and emotions that must be in the right place.

Treating Erectile Dysfunction

When I treat a male with ED, the first task is to be able to rule out that there are any physical factors contributing to his problem. I want to make sure the physical causes mentioned previously are not present. Usually, I want him to have had a recent physical with his physician and been given a clean bill of health.

In the past, I started treating the male and his partner using the sex therapy process I learned indirectly from Masters and Johnson. Since 1998, I have tried recommending the use of a medication called Viagra to help cure erectile dysfunction. Viagra, Cialis, and Levitra are the trade names used for the three medications commonly prescribed for ED. The difference in these medications is the time they take to affect the body.

Viagra was originally developed by British scientists and then brought to market by the U.S.-based pharmaceutical company, Pfizer. It acts by inhibiting cGMP-specific phosphodiesterase type 5 (PDE5), an enzyme that promotes degradation of cGMP, which regulates blood flow in the penis.(11)

Some sex therapists and researchers believe that a large placebo effect occurs when men take Viagra. This not to say that there isn't a definite physiological impact when used, but there is a major psychological component as well. When a male with ED believes that taking a pill will render him erect, his performance anxiety is reduced, which, in turn, will allow him to relax and thus sexually perform. ED medication has also been found to have a placebo effect on women.

A study done in 2007 reports on women who suffer from sexual dysfunction problems, including difficulty with arousal and orgasms. In the study, all the women underwent an eight-week trial with a placebo.

They concluded that "not surprisingly, most of the women responded extremely positively to the placebo. I say not surprisingly because the reality is that this study reflects the findings of a number of other well-received studies. One compelling result in this particular study is that researchers found a heavy correlation between the rate of sexual improvement experienced by women, and tangible factors such as their age, and length of relationship. This suggests that environmental factors may have a strong impact on the effectiveness of placebo treatments."(12)

Some people believe that the ED medication can increase sex drive, which improves sexual performance, or permanently increases penis size. Studies on the effects of Viagra when used recreationally are limited, but suggest that it has little effect when used by those not suffering from erectile dysfunction.

A male's female partner sometimes takes it personally that her lover has to take a pill in order to be sexually aroused by her. She reacts with anger and hurt, that she isn't good enough to turn him on. She has to understand that his lack of responsiveness is more a matter of biology and not so much about her sexual attractiveness. Also, if she can get her sexual self-esteem out of the picture, she will be a major beneficiary in her partner's ability to perform.

The Psychological Approach

If a male patient has no major physical conditions that would contribute to having ED and has taken ED medications that are not effective in resolving the problem, then I take the more traditional approach to treating the ED problem.

The first thing I do is to take an extensive sexual history of the man's past. I want to determine the psychological environment in which the problem first occurred. I begin with questions like, "How did you feel emotionally with the woman you were with? Were you anxious or angry? Did you trust her?"

If he is married, I try to get an idea of how he feels about his marriage in general. I am trying to discover what emotional conditions for adequate sexual functioning were not being met for this particular patient.

Often, when erection difficulties are the presenting problem, the real problem is a relationship issue. Consider the example of Frank and Mary.

Frank and Mary don't spend much time communicating intimately. When they do, they end up yelling at each other and then not speaking to each other for days afterward.

Because they aren't emotionally close, Frank wants to make love to his wife to bridge the gap. When they do engage sexually, usually Mary just goes through the motions with very little feeling. When Frank becomes aware of Mary's attitude while they are making love, he loses his erection and becomes upset with himself. He then decides that he needs to go to see a sex therapist for his "problem."

In the case of a couple like Mary and Frank, therapy centers on the relationship between the two, rather than just on Frank. It is imperative that their relationship outside the bedroom be intimate enough for there to be an atmosphere in which they are relaxed and comfortable emotionally during sexual involvement.

Marital therapy often helps couples like Frank and Mary to open up their verbal communication on an emotional level in a constructive manner, in a way that brings them more intimacy, as opposed to distance.

In the case of a man who isn't in a monogamous relationship, we need to discover what his conditions for adequate sexual functioning are. Once these conditions have been defined, then it is a matter of pinpointing the specific ones that aren't being met. No matter how much ED medication a male takes, if his psychological conditions such as trust and emotional intimacy are not being met, or if he has locked or repressed resentments, the medication won't be effective. In order for these medications to be effective, a male must be in a relaxed, erotic environment.

After we have looked at whether his conditions are being met, the next step is to see if the situation he is in can be changed and, if not, to help him understand why he is unable to function sexually given the circumstances.

Breaking the Vicious Circle of Disappointment

Once the conditions for adequate sexual functioning have been met, the next therapeutic task is to break the goal-oriented loop. This loop pattern was best illustrated with the previous case example of Jack and Sue and the psychological trap that Jack fell into once he lost his erection for the first time. If I were working with this couple in sex therapy, or with any couple with the same issues, the first thing I would do is make sexual intercourse off limits.

Some patients react to this directive with a sigh of relief because it removes the pressure to perform and to get an erection. Within sex therapy, the patient is able to let go of working at trying to achieve an erection because he is given instructions to focus his source of pleasure on everything but his penis. Refer to Chapter Twelve for more details on this step in the therapeutic process.

Once free of the goal of achieving and maintaining an erection, the man can simply focus on the pleasure of touching his partner or her touching him in an erotic context. Guess what happens then? He often gets an erection.

Usually, once he gets his first erection in a long time, he immediately wants to have intercourse with his partner, and to hell with what the therapist said. He acts as if he may never have another erection again. But in his hurried, pressured attempt to achieve his goal of intercourse, he stops experiencing the pleasure of the moment and becomes focused on penetration and what his penis is doing. As a result, he loses his erection, and again becomes angry and frustrated with himself—which only depresses him and reduces his testosterone levels, hampering his ability to achieve and maintain an erection on a physiological level.

Usually, when this experience is reported back to me in therapy, the patient is ashamed and embarrassed for not following the doctor's orders. I tell him that it's great that he got an erection, but that I want him to realize what happens when he starts trying to force his experience. He can get lots of erections, but that doesn't mean he has to do anything with them. There are more where this came from, so he can relax and enjoy the pleasure of the moment. I want the patient to feel so confident with getting an erection that in essence he can ignore it when he gets one—it is no big deal.

Erections normally rise and subside while one is involved sexually. As a man becomes more mature, he becomes more subject to distractions that might temporarily cause him to lose his erection. As Michael Castleman states in his book, *Sexual Solutions*, "The trick to raising a fallen erection is to relax and ask for some stroking that arouses you. Lost erections tend to stay lost when men get upset, order them to happen again, or berate their lovers for not being sexy enough to keep them hard."(13)

Some men who come to therapy because of erection difficulties respond differently when I tell them they are not to have intercourse for a while. Instead of being relieved, they get angry and defensive. They say things like, "I thought we were here for sex therapy! If we can't have sex, then what's the point?"

It is difficult for them to see that sex is more than intercourse. This is also an understandable reaction to having someone dictate the way they should behave sexually. The man in this case is having a hard time letting go of control and being vulnerable in the therapeutic process.

The awareness experience described in Chapter Seven can be useful in breaking the goal-orientation process. This helps the patient learn to keep his focus on the pleasure of the moment, instead of thinking about whether or not he is getting an erection. This kind of thinking takes him out of the pleasure of the moment and causes him to lose his erection.

Once a client is able to experience erections confidently through means of stimulation other than intercourse, then it is time to include intercourse. At this point, I tell the patient that it is normal for him to have erections that vary in intensity or hardness. This is because the sexual response cycle has various stages. If he happens to lose his erection during sexual arousal, it just means that his sexual arousal has dropped off; it is no big deal. He knows that he is able to get erections because he has in the past. It is just a matter of focusing his attention on the pleasure of the moment and on something that excites him sexually about his partner or what she could do to give him more pleasure.

It is important for a man who has problems with erections to remember that he has alternatives to stimulating his partner with his penis. The issues here are similar to those that occur with men who have premature ejaculation. Understanding that he has options in sexual stimulation results in a great decrease in psychological pressure about his ability to get an erection. This, in turn, enables him to relax if he happens to lose his erection while having intercourse.

If he wants to, he can pleasure his partner using his hands or mouth, or she may want to start pleasuring him. In any case, the goal is not to get an erection. The focus is sexual pleasure. When the man's attention is directed toward sexual pleasure in general, he will probably get an erection, and if he so desires, he may want to resume having intercourse. All of these sexual interactions are based on the assumption that they are acceptable to his partner.

To digress for a moment, I have encountered the belief that somehow a male should get an erection just by being with his partner, without any physical stimulation. This may be the case when the couple is first dating and there is a great deal of newness to their sexual interaction. Just the anticipation of a possible sexual encounter would be psychologically stimulating enough for a male to experience an erection.

This type of seemingly automatic erection is great when it happens, but to believe that an erection must or should always occur in this way is unrealistic. After a man has been involved with his partner for a period of time, he becomes fairly familiar with her body and her responses. I'm not suggesting that they aren't sexually attracted any more after the novelty wears off, merely that there won't be the same kind of automatic erection, especially if there is a degree of fatigue.

Many men believe that their penises should be able to rise to erection on command. In pornography on the Internet, men usually present their lovers with fully formed, throbbing erections from the moment they remove their clothes. What the man who has formed his sexual beliefs from porn on the Internet should remind himself is that he does not know what went on to stimulate that erection while the camera was off.

To summarize: The primary therapeutic strategy in treating erection difficulties is to break the vicious goal-oriented loop. Once this has been accomplished, the patient will start to develop a greater confidence in his erection capacity. He will, through the treatment process, have a better intellectual understanding about his own sexuality, free of the misconceptions that set him up for sexual problems. If he loses his erection, panic won't set in because of what he has learned. Instead, he will refocus his attention on the moment and on experiencing the erotic pleasure he is receiving; an erection will naturally result.

The preceding discussion is based on the assumption that the man's more deep-seated psychological issues associated with his ability to experience an erection have been sufficiently resolved. Likewise, any relationship issues between the male and his partner must also have been worked through, so that a loving condition exists between them.

Premature Ejaculation

Of all the male dysfunctions, premature ejaculation, also known as PE, is the most common in men younger than 40 years, with 30–70 percent of males in the United States affected to some degree at one time or another.(14) Given all the media attention that ED gets, you would think that it's the most common problem. PE occurs in men of all socioeconomic levels, so no one is exempt from the possibility of developing this problem.

The term premature ejaculation implies that we know the right time for an ejaculation to occur. But when is ejaculation premature? Is it premature if it occurs before the man enters his partner's vagina? Ten seconds after he enters? Two minutes? Ten minutes? An hour? Of course, any answer would be arbitrary. Obviously, before entering the vagina would be premature, but beyond that it is best to get the clock out of the picture.

Masters and Johnson define premature ejaculation as the inability to delay ejaculation long enough for the woman to have an orgasm at least 50 percent of the time.(15) According to their definition, the man's prematurity is connected to his partner's opportunity or ability to experience orgasm. But what if she isn't orgasmic through intercourse? The man could last for an hour, and he still would be considered premature by their definition.

After Shere Hite came out with her research on the female orgasm in her book, *The Hite Report*, she reported that between a very large percentage of women are not orgasmic with vaginal stimulation only.(16) According to Planned Parenthood statistics, as many as one in three women have trouble reaching orgasm when having sex. And as many as 80 percent of women have difficulty with orgasm from vaginal intercourse alone.(17)

So, if a man is having intercourse with a woman who is unable to reach orgasm through intercourse alone, he would be considered premature, no matter how long he lasted.

Dr. Helen Singer Kaplan defines premature ejaculation as the absence of voluntary control. That is, the man has little or no control over when he ejaculates. My concept of premature ejaculation is similar to Dr. Kaplan's. I define premature ejaculation as when a male feels he has no control over his ejaculatory response. It's more about the sense of control than time on the clock. A male who has PE feels as if he is on a runaway train that can't be stopped.

Reactions to Premature Ejaculation

The initial reaction to having PE is feeling embarrassment and shame. The man feels as though he has failed and feels very inadequate as a lover. He has let his lover down and is upset with himself. He harbors a great sense of guilt because he got satisfaction—i.e., an orgasm—but he knows that his lover didn't, because he came before she had a chance. He probably believes that the only way to give his lover an orgasm is through vaginal intercourse.

The main overriding emotion for a male with premature ejaculation is a lot of anxiety. This high level of anxiety related to his lack of control over his speed of ejaculation prohibits his ability to relax and be present with his and his partner's sexual experience in the moment. It is impossible for a man to be sensitive and responsive to his partner while he is worried that he might come too fast. His partner may react to his insensitivity and take it personally and feel rejected and hurt, besides experiencing a great deal of sexual disappointment. It would be difficult for a male with PE to be in touch and aware of his own sexual experience in this situation because he is so full of anxiety about his lack of ejaculatory control that he has a difficult time enjoying the pleasure of the moment. Sometimes, he is so worried about his speed of ejaculation that he isn't able to achieve an erection and develops a secondary problem of ED.

Common Causes

As with most of the sexual dysfunctions, PE can appear as either a chronic or acute problem. When premature ejaculation has been a long-term problem, its roots nearly always go back to the man's early sexual development. After listening to the sexual histories of hundreds of males with premature ejaculation problems, I have noticed a common pattern.

A man's first ejaculations usually occur through masturbation. For the man who has PE, these early experiences were filled with guilt and anxiety. He was usually in a hurry, trying to get it over as quickly as possible so as not to get caught. He could never simply relax and enjoy the experience for as long as he wanted to pleasure himself.

When he first experienced intercourse, the same conditions existed. Perhaps he was having intercourse with a girl in the back seat of a car, or in his or her parents' living room. Again, the experience was pervaded by the constant fear of being caught. At the same time, since he didn't know much about what to do sexually, he felt nervous or anxious. He has come to associate fear and anxiety with sex, and premature ejaculation is the natural physical manifestation of these emotions.

Now, he's on his honeymoon with his new wife. He feels anxious again. He wants the experience to be memorable; therefore, he feels pressure to perform. He cannot relax. Both because of his lack of confidence based on his past sexual experiences and because of the anxiety arising from the present situation, he ejaculates prematurely. He is out of control. Gradually, his prematurity becomes a consistent problem with his new wife. He becomes frustrated and develops a sense of inadequacy as a lover and tends to lose interest in sex altogether.

The pattern worsens the longer it continues. And this is true for nearly all sexual dysfunctions, whether male or female related. The problem almost never takes care of itself over time.

The Vicious Circle of Premature Ejaculation

Premature ejaculation, like the other sexual dysfunctions, is a vicious circle. The circle goes something like this: when he knows that he is going to be sexual with his partner, the man starts thinking about whether he will be able to last very long. This could, for example, be at lunchtime before the evening in question. When he begins thinking about the upcoming event and his "performance," his anxiety begins to build. During the afternoon, he is able to repress his anxiety somewhat by concentrating on his job, but (as we have seen) repressed emotions don't simply go away. When he comes home from work and sees his partner, he thinks again about the sexual experience to come later that evening and feels more anxiety.

By the time he and his partner are in bed together, he has created a great deal of performance anxiety for himself. When he does begin to interact sexually, his thoughts are centered mainly on not ejaculating. Having accumulated during the day, his anxiety is now heightened by the circumstance of the moment, making him extremely tense. Since he cannot relax and enjoy the pleasure of the moment, he ejaculates prematurely, which confirms his earlier fears, reinforcing his insecurity.

The person suffering from PE becomes goal oriented. His goal is to not ejaculate prematurely. But the more goal oriented he becomes, the less he is able to focus on the pleasure of the moment, and so he creates more anxiety for himself. The more anxiety he feels, the more apt he is to ejaculate prematurely, which causes him to become even more goal oriented, and so on, until he gives up and doesn't want to be sexual at all and loses his desire.

Explanations for Premature Ejaculation

The traditional psychoanalytic explanation for premature ejaculation is that the man has repressed intense, but unconscious, sadistic feelings toward women. These feelings probably have their origin in his relationship with his mother. The unconscious purpose of ejaculating quickly is to defile and soil the woman and deprive her of her own pleasure. While this explanation may be true in some cases, it most definitely is not true for the majority of men who love their wives and don't have sadistic feelings toward women; their speed of ejaculation is just out of their control.

Some therapists see premature ejaculation as an unconscious weapon in a couple's struggle for power or control. The woman wants her partner to postpone his ejaculation, so that she can experience more pleasure. The man, as a way of getting back at her for something she has done outside the bedroom, rebels and ejaculates quickly. Again, this explanation may be accurate in some instances, but not in most. Whatever the general explanation for PE (and I tend to agree with Masters and Johnson, who ascribe it to stress during the male's initial sexual experiences), one thing is clear: it is rarely caused by a physical condition. It almost always has to do with the individual's thinking and subsequent emotions, and his experience of high anxiety as it relates to his sense of having no control over his sexual response.

Unmet Conditions

Some men experience sexual dysfunctions such as premature ejaculation acutely only in certain situations with certain sexual partners. For them, it is likely that their conditions for functioning sexually are not being met. As Bernie Zilbergeld puts it in *Male Sexuality*, "A condition is anything at all that makes a difference to you sexually. It can involve your physical and emotional state, how you feel about your partner, what you think you can expect from her, the type of stimulation you want, the setting you are in, or anything else. A condition is anything that makes you more relaxed, more comfortable, more confident, more sexual, more open to your experience in a sexual situation."(18)

In most cases of premature ejaculation associated with specific situations, the initial problem is that the man's conditions are not being met. Here are a few examples, showing the sorts of conditions that can be contributing factors.

John is 35 and has been married for ten years. During this time, he has learned from experience that when his wife, Sue, does things that irritate him, it is better to repress his resentments. He has learned this because whenever he does try to communicate his anger, she blows up and withdraws emotionally until he apologizes for upsetting her.

When they make up after one of these verbal transgressions, Sue always wants to make love. Wanting to please her, he consents, even though he is still feeling resentful over their argument. When they have intercourse, John ejaculates quickly, which makes Sue even more upset with him. John, in turn, feels inadequate as a lover and as a man.

What are the conditions that are not being met for John? The most obvious one is that he requires an acceptable level of emotional comfort. How can John expect to be emotionally comfortable with someone toward whom he has a great deal of anger? It is very difficult to be sexually intimate with someone you resent at the same time.

This is exactly what John's penis is trying to tell him. If John's penis could talk, it would probably say something like, "You want me to go inside this woman you are angry with and give her pleasure? You've got to be kidding! You might be able to force me in there, but I'm going to get out as fast as I can."

A penis's behavior is often linked to its owner's true feelings. The key to correcting most sexual problems is to learn what the message is, so that it can be communicated in a better way. Too often, a man knows what the message is, but tries to ignore it because it isn't flattering to his sexual self-image.

Another example is Steve, who is 32 and recently divorced from his first wife of 12 years. Not having had many sexual relationships prior to marriage, Steve was really looking forward to dating. Sex hadn't been very good or frequent in his marriage, but he had experienced no sexual problems.

After dating for a while, he had his first sexual opportunity since his divorce. Though he was excited about this opportunity, when the magic moment arrived, he became extremely nervous and afraid that somehow he wouldn't be good enough. He wanted to impress his new lover with how proficient he was at lovemaking, but he didn't have any idea of the kinds of things she liked sexually.

As a consequence of his emotional state at the time, from his viewpoint, Steve had ejaculated prematurely. He felt embarrassed and inadequate as a lover and wanted another chance to prove himself.

The next time he went out with his new woman friend, he thought about how he wasn't going to ejaculate so quickly. In fact, he thought about it the whole day before going out with her. He thought that perhaps if he thought about his job while making love, it might make him last longer so he could satisfy his partner thoroughly. Again, Steve felt anxious when they went to bed together. While they were making love, he tried to think of work, but again, he ejaculated very quickly. On the way home that night, he was angry with himself and subsequently became depressed. He became so afraid that he didn't ask the woman out again.

What sexual condition was not being met for Steve? One important requirement for a good, pleasurable sexual experience is the ability to relax. Obviously, this is something that Steve couldn't do in either situation with his new lover. He was trying to live up to unrealistic expectations that he had imposed on himself. He was trying to be perfect—which will give anyone a load of anxiety and create tension and the inability to relax because perfection doesn't exist with humans.

One important condition that Steve needs to have met, and one that is fairly universal, is the absence of judgment. In Steve's case, the judgment wasn't coming from his lover, but from himself. He was furious with himself for ejaculating quickly, which only made his condition worse. He needed to learn to accept that, given the conditions, his sexual performance made sense. Accepting what is happening doesn't mean liking it, but refusal to accept it only compounds the problem.

The last condition not being met for Steve was, again, emotional comfort. Many men who have just come out of long-term relationships and find themselves newly single have problems like Steve's. In his marriage, he had been aware of no sexual difficulties; it was just that sexual activity was infrequent, especially toward the end when he didn't realize that his wife was involved with another man. He intuitively knew that something wasn't right between them, but didn't want to acknowledge that reality. But once he found out about the extramarital affair and the couple subsequently divorced, he found himself out in the singles world. He lost the psychological cocoon that his wife represented to him. Even if a husband and wife fight or are unhappy with each other, there is a certain comfort inherent in a long-term relationship, at least on a sexual level.

The problem is that Steve probably thinks, as do many men, that being emotionally comfortable isn't necessary for having a good sexual experience. For some men this may be true, but not for the majority. Steve has put himself in a situation that conflicts with his unrealistic expectations and with his own particular sexual conditions. He has a major case of cognitive dissonance, which creates anger and performance anxiety, all of which set him up for more sexual difficulty.

The Fear of Intimacy and Commitment

So far in this section, we've discussed the more immediate causes of premature ejaculation. As I mentioned, there are also many possible deep-seated causes of this problem. We cannot examine all of these, but I would like to mention one that seems to crop up frequently: the fear of intimacy.

This fear is usually unconscious, so that the individual isn't aware that it exists, or that it is getting in his way. I am often alerted to the presence of the fear of intimacy or commitment by a male patient's tendency to place great importance on the symbolic meaning of intercourse. Usually, to him it represents psychological commitment. It is really rather like the old attitude of the 1950s, which showed that when you have intercourse, it means you love the woman and you plan to marry her.

If the man fails to follow through on these expectations, then he feels he is a bad person for using his lover. He then experiences much guilt and shame. The fear and anxiety kick in when he realizes he doesn't intend to marry the woman, or he is afraid of emotional commitment and begins to panic at some level, when he starts to feel he's headed down that road.

Since the fear of intimacy and commitment is often unconscious, it may conflict with his conscious intent, which is to have intercourse with his lover. As a result of this internal conflict, he ejaculates right at the onset of intercourse or soon after penetration has occurred. He may have no difficulty sexually before intercourse because there is no conflict, but once intercourse is imminent, the conflict surfaces physically with an ejaculation that is out of control.

Treating Premature Ejaculation

Many men who experience premature ejaculation try to control their speed of ejaculation by trying all kinds of self-help methods to take their psychological and physical focus away from whatever sexual stimulation they are experiencing during the sexual act. These common-sense methods include shifting their attention to antierotic images, tensing anal muscles, biting their lips, thinking about work, sports, or politics—anything but sex.

It's as if men with PE don't care about their own sexual experience and pleasure. All they care about is controlling their speed of ejaculation for their partner's sexual pleasure. This makes sense when you know they have bought into the concept that their partner's sexual fulfillment is their responsibility. It's their job, and they want to succeed.

These self-help methods work to avoid erotic sensations, but don't solve the problem of premature ejaculation. They are effective in trying to make a male's penis an object for his female partner's sexual satisfaction, but his own sexual pleasure is minimized.

This raises an important question. Why is this man making love? Is he just there for his partner? If she just wanted a penis without any brain or emotions attached, she could masturbate. It would be a lot easier if he just gave his partner a dildo and he could just watch her satisfy herself. He is willing to turn himself into a machine just so that his partner can have an orgasm through intercourse. His partner may want to have an orgasm, but I doubt that she wants a machine for a lover.

This idea again speaks to men's objectification and goal-oriented view of the sexual experience. It is more about accomplishing the goal, rather than enjoying the pleasure of the experience and sharing an intimate emotional connection with their partner. The man is so focused on the goal of not ejaculating that he is deliberately not paying attention to the process. He is willing to do anything to reach his goal; pleasure is entirely secondary.

Gaining Control: The Stop/Start Method

Instead of trying not to have sexual feelings, I suggest an opposite tack to my patients with premature ejaculation. I suggest that the man indulge himself with sexual feelings and have confidence that he can relax in the situation, assuming that his basic sexual conditions are met. As contradictory as this may seem to the man who is suffering from premature ejaculation, this process works. It's called the stop/start method. This therapeutic approach was developed after Masters and Johnson and was far more successful than the method they used in their clinic, which was called the frenulum squeeze technique.

For the man who ejaculates prematurely, one of the more important things to understand is the point of inevitability—the point at which ejaculation becomes inevitable. No matter what a man does, he can't stop his ejaculation. One of the goals of the stop/start method is to help the premature ejaculator know when he is getting close to his point of inevitability, so that he can reduce his level of sexual stimulation. Usually, a male who suffers from premature ejaculation has no sense of when he is getting close to orgasm, and by the time he realizes this, it's too late.

The first step of the stop/start method is to have the male patient masturbate to when he thinks he is getting close to the point of inevitability. When he thinks he is getting close, he is then instructed to reduce stimulation to the point where his urge to ejaculate is gone. Once this occurs, he is then told to go back to self-stimulation, to the point where he is getting close again, and then stop. My intention as his therapist is for him to have confidence that through masturbation, he can control his speed of ejaculation and last as long as he wishes.

It is the man's sense of having no control over the timing of his ejaculation that is at the heart of the problem. The sense of having no control creates the anxiety and his inability to relax, which is crucial to being able to enjoy sexual pleasure. I am trying to give him that sense of control and mastery over his ejaculation through the stop/start method.

To give you a sense of what it feels like to be a premature ejaculator, ask yourself what it would be like to drive a car without any brakes. How would you feel? I assume that you would be scared out of your mind! You would be a nervous, anxious wreck. That is what a premature ejaculator feels like when he is involved sexually. In a sense, he is having sex with his partner without the sense of brakes—i.e., the inability to stop; this, in turn, causes him a great deal of anxiety, and he loses control.

It would be pretty difficult to enjoy a Sunday drive if you had no brakes and were out of control. This is why a male with no control of his speed of ejaculation can't really enjoy his own sexual experience. But once he has control back, it's an entirely different situation.

The next step in the therapy process is to bring his partner into the treatment. Instead of the patient masturbating to the point of inevitability, I suggest that his partner stimulate him, either manually or orally, to the level of excitement where he is getting close to the point of inevitability; then, he is to instruct her to stop stimulation. Once the urge to ejaculate is removed, she can go back to stimulating him and repeat the process, until he again feels confident that he can control his speed of ejaculation through this process of arousal.

Another key concept with the stop/start method is giving the patient permission that he can stop stimulation when he is interacting with his partner. Premature ejaculators—and many men in general—don't believe that they can stop stimulation once the sexual interaction begins. When I tell a man to stop when he is getting close, he might say, "I can't stop. She will get upset with me because I am frustrating her efforts." Again, we see the goal orientation operating in this thinking. I respond: "She will get upset if you don't stop and ejaculate in an out-of-control manner." So, giving him permission to stop is like giving the brakes back to the driver of a car that previously didn't have them. In turn, this gives the driver the ability to stop, so she can relax and enjoy the ride.

Once the patient has the confidence of control over ejaculation with his partner through oral or manual stimulation of his penis, then I suggest that they try intercourse in the same way. This is the time for the patient to learn to control the level of his sexual arousal during intercourse, by varying the type of stimulation he is receiving. He can, for example, vary the intensity of stimulation by controlling the frequency of thrusting in and out of the vagina. He can also control what areas of his penis receive stimulation by varying the positions he uses during intercourse. Usually, I suggest that his partner is in the female-astride position, with the male patient on his back. This enables him to be in a more relaxing position and allows his partner to disengage during penetration. Just as before, when he is getting close to the point of inevitability, he needs to tell her to lift off his penis and stop all stimulation until his urge to ejaculate is gone, and then they can reengage in intercourse. Now, he has control during intercourse through the stop/start method.

Just like the driver of a car who knows he has brakes and may not need to use them, he can relax as he drives because if he needs them to stop, the brakes are there when needed. This is the same with a premature ejaculator giving himself permission to stop stimulation when he is getting close to the point of inevitability. He can relax sexually, which then allows him to enjoy the experience, and if he is getting too close, he can slow it all down by reducing the stimulation of his penis.

Another sexual belief that causes performance anxiety for the premature ejaculator (or anyone else for that matter) is the idea that the only right or normal way that a woman can experience an orgasm is through penile stimulation while having intercourse. Obviously, this attitude puts a great deal of pressure on a man to be able to postpone his ejaculation. If he believes he has no option in satisfying his partner other than to use his penis, he will feel a lot of anxiety—at least until he has considerable confidence in controlling his ejaculation.

Even if a man does have confidence, limiting his options could produce a rather monotonous sexual experience for both partners, thus causing the relationship to become boring.

Retarded Ejaculation

The last male sexual dysfunction that I have encountered in my clinical experience is called retarded ejaculation, or RE. This problem is fairly rare compared to the other two previously discussed dysfunctions. Sometimes, this dysfunction is called delayed ejaculation or inhibited ejaculation.

RE becomes a problem for a male when he has little difficulty obtaining and maintaining an erection and is responsive to erotic stimulation. His problem is that he is unable to ejaculate, even though he wants to have an orgasm. RE sometimes can be a mild condition, where a man can still experience an orgasm through vaginal stimulation, but only under certain conditions. A more moderate case of RE is where a man can't ejaculate through vaginal stimulation, but can through oral or manual stimulation. The most severe case of RE occurs when a man can ejaculate only when he is alone, or he just cannot ejaculate at all.

Causes

Physiological factors rarely play a role in with this dysfunction, but in some cases, they can be a factor. Possible causes include something called hypogonadism, where the testes are not producing enough testosterone, thyroid disorders, pituitary disorders, surgery of the prostate, and drug and alcohol use. In most cases, the issue isn't physiological, but psychological in nature. One such cause is the fear of letting go or becoming vulnerable to one's partner. This unresolved fear might have its roots in childhood, when it manifested itself as a fear of being abandoned by his primary love object at that time, his mother.

In adulthood, the unconscious or sometimes conscious fear comes up again in the form of anxiety during sexual intercourse. The man is already vulnerable, and to let go and ejaculate would put him in an even more vulnerable condition. Fearing this, he becomes anxious and is unable to let go sufficiently to enjoy the pleasure he is receiving to allow him to experience an orgasm and ejaculate.

Some men have difficulty ejaculating because they are so busy trying to please their partner that they don't pay enough attention to their own sexual needs. A man may focus on his partner's pleasure, not his own. He pays attention to his own just enough to get an erection (which is, of course, essential in his mind for giving his partner the "right" form of pleasure), and then he shifts his focus to watching and monitoring the partner's reactions while having intercourse.

As a result, this individual experiences the two major sources of sexual anxiety at the same time: an excessive need to please, and being a sexual spectator from a judgmental point of view. It's no wonder that he is unable to relax and enjoy his sexual experience enough to ejaculate.

Once his partner has been sexually satisfied with as many orgasms as she needs, then she wants him to have an orgasm. The couple's mental focus now turns to producing an orgasm for him. Now, he feels pressured to reach a climax. He becomes anxious and unable to experience much sexual pleasure and is therefore unable to ejaculate.

In some cases, retarded ejaculation is a symptom of a power struggle in the relationship. Consider, for example, the case of Joan and Bill. They have been married for 17 years. Joan would describe Bill as a very nice guy. He has never gotten angry with her, at least not as far as she could tell. He has always done what she wanted, without much conflict. Their only problem is that when they have intercourse, he rarely ejaculates. This has been a long-term problem, but it occurs more frequently now. At first, Joan was sympathetic, but now she has become upset and regards the problem as a form of rejection.

In this example, Bill is expressing his resentments toward Joan by holding back. It is a passive-aggressive behavior that he probably is not conscious of and doesn't understand. He too wonders why his body won't cooperate and allow him to give his wife what she wants, as he does in all other aspects of their relationship.

Again, we find the penis speaking the truth about how he feels emotionally. If Bill's penis could speak, it would probably say, "I'm not going to ejaculate into this woman and give her emotional satisfaction. I have so much resentment toward her because you won't express your anger about the things that bother you. Bill, you are afraid of her. Well, I'm not, and I know that it really drives her nuts when I don't come in her during intercourse. Until you express your anger up front, I'm not going to ejaculate inside her." Understand that this dialogue is occurring at an unconscious level inside Bill's mind; consciously, he is probably unaware of this internal conflict.

An Erotic Conflict

A common erotic conflict that results in retarded ejaculation occurs when a couple is trying to have a baby, but the male partner isn't able to ejaculate frequently enough while having intercourse to conceive a child. The husband in this case tells his wife that he wants to have a child, but physically keeps experiencing the problem of RE. Again, his unconscious is using his penis as its mouthpiece. Unconsciously, this man is afraid to let this fact come to the surface, for fear of the impact it would have on his wife and their marriage, given the fact that she wants a child very badly.

This man is responding to an unconscious message that tells him not to ejaculate enough to impregnate his wife. As long as it's unconscious, he doesn't have to take responsibility for his action or deal with the conflict because it's his body that is rebelling, not his conscious self.

The last common erotic conflict that causes retarded ejaculation is when a male has experienced some type of sexual trauma in conjunction with a sexual experience. The trauma could have taken place either during the individual's childhood such as being molested or abused then, or during more recent times.

In one common form of childhood trauma, the man grows up in a very religious family that regards sex as evil and dirty. The trauma itself occurs when this attitude is enforced during adolescence, with constant watchdog behavior on the part of the parents as to what their son is doing sexually. When they discover any kind of sexual activity like masturbation while looking at a magazine or the Internet, or kissing a girl, they punish him severely, probably both physically and emotionally. For a young, developing adolescent who is very vulnerable about his sexuality, this type of experience can leave a major scar that can last for a long time. This same type of trauma persists if the male patient was molested as a child, or was the victim of some other act of sexual abuse.

As a result of this childhood trauma, a man can have an internal psychological conflict about his sexual feelings. The adult part of him wants to be sexual with his wife, but when he becomes aroused, the little boy in his psychological makeup feels anxiety and guilt. This internal conflict manifests itself in the form of retarded ejaculation. He is able to get an erection—representative of the adult in him—but the anxious, guilt-ridden child within causes him to have difficulty in ejaculating.

Emotional traumas that occur later in life can have a similar effect, as in the case of the man who catches his girlfriend or wife in bed with another man, or whose wife tells him that she is involved with another man. Often, the man in the latter situation wants to be sexually involved with his spouse in an attempt to hang on to her. He regards sex as a form of reassurance that his wife still loves him. The man in this case usually feels guilty about not being there for his wife, both emotionally and sexually. Now that his marriage is threatened by another man, he is trying to compensate for his neglect.

When he is sexually involved with his partner under these circumstances, the man may experience some form of sexual dysfunction such as retarded ejaculation. Once again, we have an individual who has an internal psychological conflict related to his sexual feelings. One part of him wants to be sexually close because of his fears of abandonment, and he sees sex as a way of hanging on to his partner. Another part is afraid to let go and to become vulnerable because of his fear of getting hurt by his wife due to her lack of emotional commitment to their relationship. As a result of the conflict, the man may be able to get an erection, but is unable to ejaculate through intercourse. The idea of relaxing and "letting go" creates too much anxiety and fear, which gets in the way sexually.

A New Cause of Retarded Ejaculation

Gary Wilson, a contributor to the website, *Your Brain on Porn*, wrote that many porn users report that delayed ejaculation was a precursor to their erectile dysfunction. Years of porn use can cause a variety of symptoms, which, when examined, lie on a spectrum. It's likely that a combination of "death-grip" masturbation methods, desensitization of the reward circuitry, and sensitized addiction pathways are behind these various symptoms, including the following:

- Masturbating without porn is "unsatisfying," or difficult
- Earlier genres of porn are no longer "exciting"

- Experiencing greater sexual excitement with porn than with a partner
- Decreasing sensitivity of penis
- Declining sexual arousal with sexual partner(s)
- Losing erection while attempting penetration
- Little or no stimulation from penetrative sex
- Needing to fantasize to maintain erection or interest with sexual partner
- Can't ejaculate (or perhaps maintain erection) with oral sex or intercourse(19)

The obvious treatment for this problem would be to quit Internet porn cold turkey. If a male is addicted to this type of sexual stimulation, then he will require treatment for his addiction.

Treating Retarded Ejaculation

The treatment for retarded ejaculation usually occurs on two levels. The first level involves the resolution of the inner conflict that the retarded ejaculation represents. The key to this process is to help the patient first realize that the inner conflict exists and to help him talk about the issues he is struggling with. This realization process is extremely powerful, and in some cases, eliminates the sexual problem entirely.

At the same time the patient and I are working on this realization, we also attempt to break the vicious circle of goal orientation. Typically, the patient creates a great deal of anxiety within himself, knowing that he will soon be involved in sexual intercourse and worrying about whether he will be able to ejaculate. By the time he is involved with intercourse, he is mentally so uptight that he is unable to let go, and therefore experiences retarded ejaculation. This again negatively reinforces his sexual experience so he loses his confidence and will be more anxious next time he is sexually involved. This pattern is played out over and over, to the point where the individual wants to avoid sex entirely.

As with the other sexual dysfunctions, the way to break the goal-orientation loop therapeutically is to take the patient's goal away through the sex therapy process. This is done by setting limits on his sexual activity. This forces him to concentrate on the present and less on what lies down the road, thus abating his anxiety.

If the patient's dysfunction is related to some past emotional trauma, then the treatment follows a desensitization process, where the patient is taken psychologically back to the event that produced the trauma. The idea is to help the patient express the emotions that he is still repressing related to the trauma. Once the situation is emotionally diffused, then the present-day sexual event will no longer trigger unresolved emotions from the past traumatic experience, and the patient will be free to experience and enjoy the events of the moment for what they are: a pleasurable event.

Works Cited

1. Zilbergeld, Bernie. The New Male Sexuality. New York: Bantam Books, 1992.
2. Masters, William, & Johnson, Virginia. Human Sexual Inadequacy. Toronto and New York: Bantam Books, 1970.
3. Annals of Internal Medicine, Aug. 5, 2003.
4. Zilbergeld, Bernie. The New Male Sexuality. New York: Bantam Books, 1992.

5. http://www.webmd.com/erectile-dysfunction/guide/ed-diabetes
6. http://www.prnewswire.com/news-releases/testosterone-therapy-a-misguided-approach-to-erectile-dysfunction-ed-159545365.html
7. http://www.askmen.com/dating/love_tip_250/286c_love_tip.html
8. http://www.sharecare.com/health/alcohol-and-health/alcohol
9. http://www.everydayhealth.com/erectile-dysfunction/why-boozing-can-be-bad-for-your-sex-life .aspx
10. www.askman.com/lovetip
11. http://en.wikipedia.org/wiki/Sildenafil
12. http://www.placeboeffect.com/erectile-dysfunction-a-placebo-cure/
13. Castleman, Michael. Sexual Solutions. New York: Simon & Schuster Touchstone Books, 1980.
14. http://emedicine.medscape.com/article/435884-overview
15. http://www.bostonmedical.com.co/content/rapid-ejaculation-review-nosology-prevalence-and-treatment
16. Hite, Shere. The Hite Report: A National Study of Female Sexuality. New York: Seven Stories Press, 1976.
17. http://www.womansday.com/sex-relationships/sex-tips/10-surprising-facts-about-orgasms-111985
18. Zilbergeld, Bernie. The New Male Sexuality. New York: Bantam Books, 1992.
19. http://www.yourbrainonporn.com

11

Sexual Dysfunctions

Causes and Treatment for Women

Initially, my clinical experience treating female sexual dysfunctions was usually done in the presence of a female co-therapist. We would work as a team with a couple. Most of my communication was with the male patient, while my co-therapist would interact with the female patient. As my sex therapist experience continued, it became financially difficult for a couple to afford two therapists' fees at the same time. So, I dealt with couples where a male sexual dysfunction was the presenting problem, and if a female dysfunction was the presenting problem, I would refer the couple to a female sex therapist. The information in this chapter comes mainly from my academic experience and from my early co-therapy history.

The Issue of Frigidity

Before and after the work of Masters and Johnson, the label of frigidity was used as a catchall phrase for all types of female sexual dysfunctions. Frigidity could refer to all forms of inhibition of sexual response, ranging from total lack of response and erotic feelings to minor degrees of orgasmic inhibition. The implication from this word is that the woman who suffers from sexual inhibition is somehow cold and hostile toward men.

"Many clinicians now regard frigidity to be a sexist term that places the blame on the woman herself rather than on her sociocultural milieu, emotional experiences, or health status, all of which can contribute to sexual nonresponsiveness.

"The term frigidity continues to be used in everyday language, commonly as an insult or derogatory term for women who are unaffectionate or are seen as sexually nonresponsive. Very likely the term is most frequently used to explain lack of interest or rejection by a woman who originally was of interest to the person making the insult.

"Female sexual dysfunction—which has replaced frigidity as a diagnostic category in psychiatry and psychology—refers to the inability of a woman to function adequately in terms of sexual desire, sexual arousal, orgasm, or in coital situations."(1)

I think frigidity is a confusing label and should be junked. The fact is that many women who get labeled as frigid or have a female sexual dysfunction are frequently warm and responsive to sexual stimulation, but maybe not in their current relationship.

In all of my years of therapy, I don't think I have seen what I would call a sexually frigid woman. Of course, I have worked with women who weren't interested in sex, but I wouldn't consider them to be cold. On the contrary, they may have been "hot"—with anger, resentment, and hurt. From the outside, you couldn't tell that they were experiencing these emotions, but after I talked to them about their relationship and their lover, it became clear how angry and resentful they were. In the beginning of their relationship, when they experienced resentments related to incidents that occurred, they repressed these emotions because they were afraid to openly communicate their feelings. They were afraid that their lover would judge them and discount or invalidate their emotions. They also didn't want to be seen as a bitch or someone who wasn't "nice."

In a way, the so-called frigid woman has to construct a psychological wall to contain her emotions of anger, resentment, and hurt. As the relationship continues over time, more and more resentment and anger are created, so the woman has to build an even thicker wall to contain all of her anger. Of course, the wall would preclude any intimacy, affection, and sexual interaction.

As a result of this defensive psychological wall, this woman is judged as being frigid because of her inability to experience intimacy. When you get close to her wall, it may seem cold, but behind the wall she has a very hot core of resentment and anger. Her fear is that her wall will crack and all her anger will be released and destroy her relationship, just like the walls of a nuclear reactor when all the radioactivity is released into the atmosphere, destroying everything around it. The sad reality is that by trying to protect her relationship in this way, she most likely will eventually lose it because of the lack of emotional and sexual intimacy.

Preorgasmic Women

The term "preorgasmic" refers to the woman who has never experienced an orgasm, at least not consciously, through any form of stimulation. Masters and Johnson refer to this type of sexual dysfunction as anorgasmia, a woman's inability to achieve an orgasm, even with adequate stimulation. The use of the word "inability" in their definition should be qualified, however. Although the term anorgasmia includes women who are medically unable to reach orgasm, the great majority of anorgasmia cases are caused by psychological, social, cultural, or relationship variables, and are therefore best treated in a sex therapy format.

Anorgasmia is usually categorized in one of three ways: as primary, secondary, or situational. Primary anorgasmia means that the diagnosed woman has never been able to achieve orgasm at any point in her life. A diagnosis of secondary anorgasmia means that the woman was consistently able to have orgasms at one time, but is no longer able to achieve them. Situational anorgasmia refers to women who can achieve orgasm in certain sexual situations, but never orgasm in other specific situations.

In 1975, sex therapist and author Lonnie Barbach published her book, *For Yourself: The Fulfillment of Female Sexuality*.(2) This was a landmark book at the time, providing help for women who weren't experiencing orgasms. At the same time, the term anorgasmic was changed to preorgasmic. Psychologically, this was a shift to a more positive tone. The label preorgasmic implies that every woman can have an orgasm: she just hasn't experienced it yet, and the condition is temporary.

During the 1970s and 1980s, being preorgasmic seemed to be the most common presenting sexual dysfunction for women. Fueled by the women's liberation movement, women wanted equality in the bedroom. Sex just wasn't for male satisfaction anymore. In a way, then, being orgasmic in their sexual relations became a political statement for some women. By the 1990s, however, it seemed that being preorgasmic seemed much less common as a sexual dysfunction. Today, I rarely see it in my clinical practice.

Why did the preorgasmic dysfunction seem to disappear? I believe its disappearance occurred because there was a cultural change in attitude that occurred during the 1970s and 1980s regarding women masturbating. It became more acceptable—almost chic—for women to masturbate just like men. The whole notion of having a "friend" in her nightstand—a vibrator—was talked about as if it was no big deal among women.

As more women became comfortable with masturbating, they learned about their own sexuality and how they could experience an orgasm. The only problem that remained was communicating this information to their partners. Many men have a problem receiving this type of communication without getting defensive because so many believe that they should know how to give their partner an orgasm without needing additional information from the partner. As discussed in Chapter Six, nothing could be further from the truth.

Other Causes of Women Experiencing Preorgasmic Difficulties

Usually, the cause of a woman not experiencing an orgasm is the inability to give herself an orgasm through masturbation, but on some occasions, there are psychological reasons that impede her orgasmic response. The following are a few that I have encountered in my practice.

One reason that reaching an orgasm for a woman may be problematic is that having one has acquired a symbolic meaning that creates a psychological conflict for the woman. She wants to let go to her lover and have a sense of abandon, but at the same time, she isn't ready to be that vulnerable. Perhaps she feels that she could only have an orgasm with someone she is in love with. Or maybe orgasm symbolizes an emotional commitment that is frightening to her because it represents a threat to her sense of autonomy.

Sometimes, the mere intensity of emotion experienced during orgasm is overwhelming to a woman. When she is close to having an orgasm, she shuts down unconsciously (or consciously) to avoid the experience. Her fear of losing control and becoming vulnerable inhibits her.

In some cases, the experience of orgasm can bring up internal conflicts in the woman about her own erotic feelings. This is called an erotic conflict. One such conflict is the Madonna-whore syndrome. Psychologically speaking, part of the woman (the so-called whore) wants to respond sexually, while the Madonna part of her is resistant. If the Madonna aspect is stronger, then the woman is unable to allow herself to experience orgasm.

Finally, a woman's hostility toward her mate may establish an involuntary over-control of her ability to experience an orgasm. Repressed resentments get in the way of experiencing full sexual potential. For her to experience an orgasm and its physical and psychological release, all her emotions will come to the surface; if she doesn't want to feel her unpleasant emotions such as hurt and anger, she blocks all emotional expression, thus blocking her erotic feelings.

All of these psychological causes of inhibited orgasmic response require treatment in the context of individual psychotherapy. But in any case, whether the woman merely needs to learn what gives her enough pleasure for orgasm, or her preorgasmic condition comes from deeper psychological blocks, once she has successfully resolved the problem, she must learn to incorporate her newly learned skills during interplay with her sexual partner. This is usually accomplished through general sex therapy approaches, which will be described later.

According to Masters and Johnson, only a small percentage of women's sexual dysfunctions are due to physical causes. The majority arise from psychological issues such as those previously discussed. However, two specific physical factors have been implicated as causes of female dysfunctions. One is the condition of clitoral adhesions, which block adequate stimulation to the clitoris. The other is inadequate pubococcygeus (PC) muscle strength and contractions.

The Dynamics or Prerequisites for the Female Sexual Response of Orgasm

The first requirement for a woman to respond sexually is that she be properly stimulated. What determines what is proper stimulation is the woman herself. Not her lover, but her, because only she knows what turns her on.

The second requirement is that a woman must be sufficiently relaxed during the sexual experience. This will enable her to respond to the stimulation she is receiving and abandon herself to the experience. If the woman is anxious about anything that is occurring in her life generally such as her children, her work, or older parents, then she most likely will not be able to relax in the moment. If she is anxious about anything going on sexually in the moment like her performance or being self-conscious about her body, this type of anxiety will block her ability to respond as well.

Even if a woman receives the right stimulation for her and she is free of anxiety and can relax, she still might not be able to respond sexually. One reason for this inhibition is that her past experiences may block her response. This could include past sexual trauma that the woman herself has blocked out of her consciousness and isn't even aware of. Often, these past experiences have to be treated through the process of clinical hypnotherapy.

The General Treatment Concepts for a Preorgasmic Woman

Some general principles are taught to women who have difficulty experiencing an orgasm. These also to apply to women in general, as they relate to their general sexuality.

The first concept is that they must take time for themselves and have patience with their sexual response. Sometimes, just the idea of a woman taking time for herself is seen as a selfish act. For a preorgasmic woman to take this time and not feel guilty is a challenge in itself. Just taking a bath for an extended period of time, where she doesn't have to give anything to anyone, can be a new experience. This can be the start to learning to give herself pleasure and create relaxation.

The next idea is to remove all thoughts that are goal oriented. She needs to learn to be in the moment, to focus on pleasure—not what *isn't* happening, but what feels good to her in that time. Taking away all the goal-oriented thoughts reduces any performance anxiety or pressure that inhibits sexual pleasure and blocks the ability to relax.

Whatever form of sexual stimulation that may work in getting her sexually excited is acceptable. There is no right way for a woman to reach an orgasm. However she gets this sexual experience is fine.

It is also acceptable to take time to reach an orgasm. There is no hurry when pleasure is involved. There is no time clock saying you must respond in a certain amount of time. However long it takes to get to the point of orgasm is the right time for that woman. If the woman puts pressure on herself to hurry up and have an orgasm, it will take her longer to come. The orgasmic response doesn't respond well to internal or external pressure.

The last general principle a preorgasmic woman needs to know is that the minute differences in the way she is touched within a sexual experience can make a major difference to her level of responsiveness. These very small differences can change from one sexual experience to another. What felt pleasurable last time may not feel good this time. These differences can change due to the woman's physiology, hormones, and her menstrual cycle, as well as her sexual mood and energy level.

Even though a woman has never experienced an orgasm, she may have a high sexual desire and fall in love, enjoy foreplay, and intercourse. A woman's experience can be conditioned easily and is vulnerable to inhibition. Usually, she isn't consciously aware of this conditioning process. One of the primary contributors to the preorgasmic condition is a woman's lack of knowledge about her own sexuality and her difficulty in taking responsibility for it; i.e., via verbal communication.

Secondary Nonorgasmic Women

In this dysfunction, a woman has had orgasms in the past through various forms of sexual stimulation, but at present is unable to do so. Usually, this condition is the result of situational factors in her life. The following are some of those factors.

Relationship Problems

In most of the secondary orgasm problems I have worked with, the woman's inability to experience orgasm stems from the emotional atmosphere between her and her partner; it is simply not conducive to the expression of erotic feelings. Generally, the woman has been repressing a great deal of resentment and anger about her mate over a number of years. When she did try to communicate these resentments, they fell on deaf ears, and as a result, she did not feel heard and understood, so the resentments weren't resolved for her. Gradually, these resentments have built up to the point that she goes numb during any sexual experience with her partner. She may have had sexual feelings in the past, but no more.

The lack of communication in one area of the relationship (in this case, her resentments) leads to an inability to communicate in other areas as well. The woman shuts off sexually because it is just too painful for her to experience any intense emotions with her partner.

In this kind of situation, I would seek to help the couple through relationship counseling before attempting sex therapy. My approach would be to help the woman express her resentments—both new and old—to her partner in a constructive way. At the same time, I would teach her partner to listen effectively, so that she is more inclined to trust that he will be there emotionally and not shut her out or down. Once she is able to trust that she can be emotionally vulnerable with her partner, she can become physically vulnerable and let go enough to have an orgasm. The resentments are then not blocking her ability to experience pleasure with her partner. This process is described in detail in my book, *Creating the Intimate Connection*.(3)

Just as the buildup of resentment toward her partner can shut down a woman's orgasmic capacity, so can a loss of trust in her partner's commitment to their relationship. Such a loss of trust usually occurs after she has become aware of an extramarital affair. Often, the wife becomes competitive, thinking she can win her husband back from his mistress and behaving in a passive manner, doing whatever he wants sexually with her. She tries to use sex as a way to hang on to him. But because of the wife's loss of trust, she is unable to become vulnerable and experience orgasm. She can be sexually involved with her husband, but can't let go, and then puts pressure on herself to be orgasmic. With this additional performance anxiety, she has created yet another barrier to orgasmic response. How long this condition exists for the woman depends on how long it takes for her to regain trust in her husband's emotional commitment to their relationship.

Obviously, this is not really a sexual problem, but a relationship issue in which the dysfunction has become the signal. From the client's point of view, the therapist should just fix her sexual problem; then all will be well. But unless the deeper relationship issues are addressed, the symptom will remain, perhaps disguised as something else.

My approach to the problem is directed toward restoring an atmosphere of trust between the couple. Once trust has been achieved, the woman's symptom of secondary nonorgasmia should disappear.

Sometimes the fact that a woman isn't having an orgasm in the moment, but has previously experienced orgasm, might indicate that her orgasmic response is caught up in a power struggle between the couple. He wants her to have an orgasm, but because she is mad about the way he treats her in general, she withholds her orgasmic response to get back at her partner for his treatment. She is willing to use her own sexual experience as a weapon to get back at her partner because she knows how important it is to her partner to give his wife an orgasm.

A woman's perception of her lover may also impede her experience of orgasm. If she perceives her lover as stupid, untrustworthy, or crude, or if she is physically afraid of him, she may have difficulty responding to him sexually no matter how beautiful his body is or how skillful he is as a lover.

Any of these aforementioned relationship issues may come into play at any time in the course of a relationship and affect a woman's orgasmic capacity with her partner.

Vaginismus

The last dysfunction we'll discuss is vaginismus. In this condition, whenever the woman attempts to engage in sexual intercourse, the entrance to her vagina closes to the point that penile penetration becomes difficult and painful, if not impossible. The muscles surrounding the vaginal entrance contract involuntarily; it is a reflex action and is not willed. In some cases, vaginismus occurs in connection with a related sexual problem known as dyspareunia, which means pain associated with intercourse. Dyspareunia and vaginismus can occur either separately or together.

Vaginismus isn't a common sexual dysfunction, but when it occurs, it is very disruptive to the individual's personal life. In some cases I have observed, the couple's marriage has been jeopardized because of the husband's frustration at the lack of sexual frequency resulting from the problem itself. This is not to say that a woman who experiences vaginismus is not sexually responsive; on the contrary: she may enjoy sexual activity and even be orgasmic, but the sexual experience doesn't involve sexual intercourse.

In this situation, sexual frequency tends to fall off because of the woman's feelings of sexual inadequacy, due in turn to her inability to have intercourse. Even though her partner may not complain, she still feels inadequate. There is an unspoken conflict not only between the couple, but also within the woman herself. Even though she enjoys sexual activity, she may avoid it because of her emotional discomfort. She finds herself in a psychological double bind. On one hand, she wants to have intimate relations with her partner and is afraid that she will lose him if she doesn't; but on the other hand, whenever they are sexually intimate, she feels a great deal of discomfort and a renewed sense of inadequacy because of her difficulty with intercourse.

Sometimes, a woman with vaginismus will seek therapy for the problem because she desires to have a child. A couple can avoid facing the vaginismus issue for years, but when the desire for children arises, the issue has to be faced. Again, this places more pressure upon the woman to have intercourse, which only adds to her problem. The only way the desire for children contributes positively to the situation is that it forces the couple to seek help.

Causes of Vaginismus

Vaginismus is an involuntary reaction to the idea of penetration or the actual experience. This reaction can occur not only with penetration related to intercourse, but also with any penetration related to the vagina, such as the insertion of a tampon.

So the question is what causes this reaction in a woman. I like to use the metaphor of what I used to go through when I got a polio vaccination as a child. In those days, the needles they used for injections weren't as fine as they are today, and the injection hurt. When I knew I was going to get a polio shot from my doctor, I would cry and beg my mom for mercy, but to no avail. When the moment came, I would tense up, and it would hurt like hell, of course. Today, when I get an injection for something, I still begin to tense up like I did as a child. Often, I am surprised that I got the shot, since I didn't feel it due to the improvement in technology. The tensing is an old conditioned response from a past experience that hasn't been totally extinguished.

In a similar way, a woman with vaginismus believes that vaginal penetration will hurt. The reason for this belief usually has to do with some experience in her past, where penetration was painful. Sometimes, penetration is associated with some type of trauma such as rape or other sexual assault or abuse. In these cases, penetration is not only physically painful, but emotionally so as well. The pain of penetration may also be associated with a painful gynecological exam when she was a teen.

In some cases, the associated pain with intercourse is related to a woman's physical self-perception that she is relatively small compared to her lover's physical size, if he is a big guy, that is, and she is a short woman in comparison. Because of this difference in body size, she might assume mistakenly that she has a small vagina and because he is much bigger in stature, he has a large penis. This distortion of belief comes from her ignorance of sexual anatomy. Vaginas and penises come in the same size, regardless of physical height and stature of the individual.

Because of her ignorance of anatomy, the woman thinks that his big penis is going to hurt. All it takes is the thought of potential pain, and she tightens up. When it occurs, intercourse hurts, which confirms her fear, even if it's based on false information.

Treating Vaginismus

In my clinical experience, these cases have been the most rewarding of all to treat. To help a married couple experience sexual intercourse for the first time without pain is quite fulfilling professionally.

The treatment of vaginismus is usually carried out on two levels. One is a straightforward behavioristic approach of physical desensitization. The other approach, which occurs at the same time, is emotional desensitization related to past traumatic experiences that triggered the dysfunction.

In the past, I was part of a therapeutic team with a female sex therapist. Generally, I would refer a woman patient who was experiencing vaginismus to the female sex therapist. It seems more appropriate for a female patient to work with a female sex therapist, given the nature of this dysfunction.

The physical desensitization process involves inserting dilators into the patient's vagina. Later, I suggested using fingers instead of plastic dilators. It seemed more personal and less mechanical. At first, the woman is instructed to insert her own fingers, one finger at first, using lubrication. The idea is for her to be in complete control of every aspect of this process. She can insert her fingers as slowly as she wants, with no pressure. After she has become comfortable with using one finger, she may use two fingers, and then three, until she is thoroughly comfortable with inserting her own fingers into her vagina. The process could take a month or longer—whatever time it takes is what works for the patient, with no pressure. This constitutes a major accomplishment for someone who has previously had difficulty inserting a tampon.

The next phase of treatment takes place in a sexual context with her partner. He is instructed to insert one of his fingers into her vagina, slowly, with lubrication. When she is comfortable with one finger, he can add another, until he reaches a total of three. As before, the duration of this process with her partner tends to vary from case to case; it simply proceeds at whatever pace the patient is comfortable with.

Once the woman is comfortable having her partner insert his fingers into her vagina and is not experiencing any pain, she is then ready for the next phase of treatment: intercourse. The couple is instructed to begin with digital insertion by the male partner. When the woman feels ready to have intercourse, the couple assumes the female-astride position; i.e., the woman on top. This position gives the woman complete control over both the degree of insertion of her partner's penis, as well as the amount and tempo of thrusting. This sense of control is essential for a woman who is afraid of having intercourse because it has always been a painful experience. Once she is able to have intercourse pain free, therapy is complete.

When I next see them in therapy, I usually don't have to ask the couple how it went the past week when they were able to have pain-free intercourse, because the smiles on their faces tell it all. They can get out the champagne and celebrate.

Works Cited

1. Sinclair Intimacy, copyright 2002. Institute,http://health.howstuffworks.com/sexual-health/sexual-dysfunction/sexual-frigidity-dictionary.htm
2. Barbach, Lonnie. *For Yourself: The Fulfillment of Female Sexuality.* New York: Signet, 1976.
3. Beaver, Daniel. *Creating the Intimate Connection.* San Diego: Cognella, 2011.

12

Specific Psychological Traps and How to Avoid Them

In this chapter, we will consider some of the sexual problems we can fall into if we are not aware of them. These are not necessarily deep-seated psychological problems, but they can be just as devastating if you are the one suffering them. If you do fall into one of these traps, the therapy prognosis is good if you seek the help of a qualified sex therapist.

Immediate Causes of Sexual Difficulties

The following are some psychological issues that can affect the sexual experience for both men and woman. The first key requirement for an individual to function sexually is that they must be able to abandon themselves to the erotic experience. They need to let go of their conscious control and some contact with their present environment. This sense of letting go of conscious control can be pretty scary for some people. I have seen many patients who cannot experience the pleasure of a professional massage for this reason.

When sexual problems occur, it often means that the couple has created an antierotic environment between them, which is destructive to the sexuality of one or both of them. Examples of an antierotic environment include situations where the couple is fighting with each other or they haven't talked to each other for a day or longer. Another instance is where either of them has been caught having an extramarital affair.

The basic psychological requirement for a great sexual experience within a committed relationship is an atmosphere of openness and trust, which allows the partners to abandon themselves to the sexual experience and be sexually vulnerable. The ability to be sexually vulnerable starts a long time before a couple is in the bedroom. The vulnerability starts on a verbal level in the living room. Hence the phrase, "You can't go from being roommates in the living room to becoming lovers in the bedroom." Vulnerability can't be turned on like a light switch.

Another key factor to experiencing satisfying sex is engaging in effective sexual behavior. Inept sexual techniques that are insensitive and ineffective impair the sexual response of women in particular and men who are 40 and older. Inadequate techniques usually stem from a lack of information and unconscious guilt and conflict dealing with sex. If you don't know what you need, you can't ask for it. So, the key is to break through the fear of rejection or abandonment for asking for what you want because you might be judged as selfish.

Anxiety: The Emotion That Blocks Sexual Pleasure

We have already seen how the expression or repression of anger can affect a couple's relationship. Another emotion that can have an equal influence is anxiety. Anxiety and sexual pleasure are natural enemies. The more anxiety a person has, the less sexual pleasure that individual will experience. Anxiety can exist in mild degrees, but if not reduced or eliminated, it can cripple an individual's sexual ability. Therefore, it is important to understand the sources of anxiety in the sexual context, so that they can be eliminated.

The Basic Causes of Sexual Anxiety

The Fear of Failure

The fear of failing to meet one's own sexual expectations or those of one's partner is a common source of anxiety. This fear of failure has become more common among both men and women as a result of the sexual revolution of the 1960s; it is also partly due to the advertising industry's relentless use of sex in marketing products coupled with increased alienation in our society, particularly among singles.

Sex has become the primary avenue for intimate communication among unmarried as well as married people. This adds tremendous psychological weight to an already sensitive aspect of people's lives by creating an expectation that each sexual encounter be incredibly fantastic. The problem is that all it really produces is anxiety. When a couple gets together sexually for the first time, they are moving into uncharted territory. Neither knows what the other likes or dislikes. They haven't built up a great deal of mutual trust, and this lack of trust inhibits their ability to be vulnerable with each other. They have made no commitment to each other, so each fears that if the sexual experience doesn't meet the other's expectations, the relationship will be terminated.

In short, in this situation, there is an expectation for sex to be terrific, but there are also all the psychological conditions that inhibit great sex from occurring. It is no wonder that the sexual experience of singles is filled with so much fear of failure. I commonly see this problem with newly divorced men who were married a long time and had felt sexually confident in their marriage. Suddenly, they find themselves in the singles world among many assertive women—or, at least, that is how it seems to them. They have left the safety of the past marriage relationship and now have to worry about their sexual ability with someone new.

Most men keep these concerns inside, which only adds to their anxiety. Their fear of failure becomes a self-fulfilling prophecy. They become so anxious that they are unable to get an erection, or they ejaculate prematurely. Once this occurs, they fall into the dysfunctional goal-oriented loop mentioned earlier, which may force them to stop dating entirely for fear of failure and embarrassment.

This same pattern of high expectation affects women as well, although in a different way. For women, the anxiety can be about how responsive they are to what their male partner is doing to them sexually. It's all about how they experience an orgasm. Many fake the response so they don't disappoint their partner. Where women really experience sexual anxiety often has more to do with how they will be judged on their physical appearance. The vulnerability of being naked can be very threatening for many women.

Another situation where the fear of failure can arise is on a couple's honeymoon night. This is especially true for a couple who abstained from intercourse during their courtship. Now, after their wedding is over and the big night has arrived, it's finally time to have intercourse. After a full day of anxiety and intense, exhausting emotions, there could hardly be a moment fraught with greater unexpressed expectations and poorer conditions! It's a setup for disappointment and failure.

Dealing with the Fear of Failure

The remedy f or this fear of failure may seem paradoxical. The person who is afraid of failure has to learn that failing is okay—in a way. Not that they should be thrilled by the idea, but they must learn not to make such a big deal of it. Failure happens. Men and women have to be shown that the psychological conditions within which they are trying to function sexually are, in fact, setting them up for failure. In fact, it couldn't happen any other way, given these conditions.

Sometimes, it's not the external antierotic conditions that cause failure so much as what goes on in our minds. An example of this is when a man who experiences the fear of sexual failure berates himself for being insecure. His internal critical parent says things like, "What's the matter with you? Be a man and stop worrying!" This, of course, only creates more anxiety. To counteract this response, the man has only to learn how to be more gentle and patient with himself, overriding the critical parent with his own adult voice. This voice can tell him that because he is human, he is will have to pay more attention to how he feels in the sexual situation. If he feels uncomfortable, he should respect that and do what he can to correct it. Without that margin of emotional comfort, he's going to be anything but a sexual hero. By respecting his emotional state and not judging how he feels, the man is loving himself: the first step to loving someone else.

Another way out of the fear-of-failure syndrome is to talk about the fear before becoming involved in a sexual experience. For example, in the case of a man who is worried about getting an erection or ejaculating prematurely, it will help if he communicates his fears to his partner before they engage in sex. This enables him to stop trying to pretend and to stop denying that he is anxious about failing. This may help him to relax. He acknowledges his fear, rather than letting it run his life. If he has a loving partner who is accepting and supportive, this course of action will be particularly helpful.

In order to do all of this, the man has to be willing to become vulnerable and let go of his macho image. If he is not willing to do so, then he is simply digging his own grave, sexually speaking. To free himself from the fear of failure, he has to give up all his unrealistic sexual expectations. He is in the same bind as women who compare their own bodies to those of women on the Internet and then feel inadequate.

Men who suffer from fear of failure have often formulated their expectation of how men should be sexually on the basis of the performance of someone in their twenties. Given that expectation, who wouldn't feel insecure? They are not allowing themselves to be human; instead, they are knocking themselves for not being the perfect machine—which, in reality, doesn't exist. The fear of failure also relates to the issue of responsibility, which we explored in Chapter Six. As we noted there, it is impossible to be responsible for someone else's sexual experience.

Some men and women—though mostly men—feel that they should be perfect in terms of how they make love to their partner. But they don't really have any extraordinary knowledge or skill that would justify this belief, and so feel they have to guard against anyone, particularly their partner, discovering this truth. (Of course, their partner knows the truth anyway.)

So, when his partner makes suggestions about ways to improve their lovemaking, the man may take it as a put-down and get defensive. If this defensive posture succeeds in warding off the partner's suggestions, the man's own sexual ignorance remains intact. He has locked himself into a tight sexual bind, resulting in fear of failure and anxiety. If left untreated, this bind can increase to a crippling level where sexual activity ceases altogether.

The way out of the bind is for the person to remove the burden of feeling sexually responsible for their partner. This is done by realizing that the best kind of lover is one who is receptive to new information about pleasuring their partner more effectively. It isn't a fault or a sign of inadequacy if one doesn't know everything to begin with.

Demand for Performance

Another source of anxiety is the demand for sexual performance. This can come from one's partner or from oneself, and it can be imagined or real. Whatever the source, a real or imagined demand for sexual performance is crippling to an individual's erotic experience.

The physiological performance most men demand from themselves is an erection. The problem with this is that an erection is an involuntary reflex; it cannot be produced on demand. Even though this is a simple physical reality, millions of men think that if they just keep pushing and trying, they will eventually get an erection. But they are often frustrated, because the more they demand an erection, the less likely they are to get one.

Once again, we find goal orientation getting in the way. The more demanding we are of ourselves sexually, the more anxiety we experience. The more anxiety we experience, the less sexual pleasure we have—and for most men, the less likely we are to have or maintain an erection.

When a man perceives this demand for performance, whether from his partner or from his own mind, he will probably abstain from all sexual contact entirely. This lack of interest can be misunderstood and labeled as a lack of sex drive, but it is really an avoidance of an uncomfortable situation. This makes complete sense. Who would want to be in a situation where there is a demand for sexual performance?

Women also find themselves in a position where there is a demand for sexual performance. One thing that is often demanded of them is the sexual response of orgasm—usually during intercourse. At times, it is not only the woman's partner who expects her to have an orgasm through intercourse, but herself as well. She feels inadequate as a woman if she doesn't come through penile-vaginal stimulation. She may also feel that she has let her lover down if she cannot perform this way, since many men feel that if they can't bring their partner to orgasm through intercourse, then they have failed.

As before, no one is responsible for a lover's sexual experience. Because of anatomical differences, sometimes it is a physical impossibility for a woman to experience orgasm with additional stimulation—she just cannot get enough physical contact on the clitoral area to experience an orgasm. It doesn't matter how good her lover is in this case because it's a matter of anatomy, not prowess. The clitoris has approximately 8,000 nerve endings and is the most sensitive part of the female body, not the vagina.

An Excessive Need to Please the Partner

This sounds like sexual heaven, to have a partner who wants to please you to the point where it becomes excessive, but it can turn into sexual hell. The definition of an excessive need to please is when the need to please becomes a compulsion to perform or to serve, not to disappoint, and can be a severe source of sexual anxiety.

Of course, there is nothing wrong with trying to please one's partner, but when this effort becomes compulsive, it can stifle the sexual experience of the overzealous pleasure provider. He or she can become so anxious about pleasing that it evolves into a sexual problem. People with this problem start worrying about their sexual performance because they don't want to disappoint their partners, either on the receiving or the giving end. And this excessive need to please the partner turns into a perceived demand for performance.

I have often seen men who have become so concerned about satisfying their partners with orgasms that their concern backfires on them. They continually ask their partners, "Did you come? Was it good? How many times?" As a result, the woman begins to feel anxious about having orgasms. "Is he keeping score?" She wants to please him, and her anxiety then inhibits her orgasmic ability. This turns rapidly into a vicious circle, and both partners become sexually frustrated.

Sometimes, a person can become so concerned with the pleasure of their partner that sexual contact becomes a job, or hard work—which is hardly the point of sexual intercourse! This problem usually occurs for men whose sexual egos rest on their ability to please their partner. They turn themselves into sexual machines whose only purpose is to please. They ignore their own pleasure, and then wonder why they are developing a certain amount of resentment toward their partners, which will interfere with their sexual desire for the partner over time.

When one or both partners has an excessive need to please the other, the sexual focus becomes thought oriented. Their thoughts are not generally erotic, but rather utilitarian, concerned only with the mechanical process of pleasing the other person.

These sorts of thoughts get in the way of the pleasure of the moment. Hence, the person becomes anxious and uptight, which defeats the initial intention. The partner can almost always read this tension, which inhibits that person's own pleasure as well.

For a man, this mental-sexual thinking might sound like this: "I can't come too fast; I've got to hold it a long time or she won't be pleased," or, "I've got to get an erection quickly or she'll think I'm not turned on by the way she looks."

The thoughts of a woman with an excessive need to please might sound something like this: "I have to hurry and have an orgasm or he will be disappointed with me," or "I can't take this much time—he is getting impatient," or, "I can't ask him to go down on me; he will be repulsed."

All these thoughts about performance take a person from focusing on what they are feeling in the moment to antierotic thoughts about performance, which take away their experience of pleasure. Some therapists call this kind of thinking and worrying "mind fucking." These thoughts sabotage an individual's sexual relationship.

Sexual Codependency

An excessive need to please can quickly turn into a codependent situation. The person who has this need tends to view their partner as someone needing help, a victim who must be taken care of from a pit of sexual frustration. The problem with being a codependent is that you take on the responsibility of solving or fixing the problem of the so-called victim. The codependent robs the victim of the chance to learn how to fix his or her own sexual problem. You can't fix someone's sexual problem; only the individual can do that—and if you try, it will backfire on you. The harder you try, the more you get frustrated, and this frustration can turn into resentment. A transformation occurs where the codependent starts out trying to be nice and helpful and then turns mean and begins to verbally attack the partner with the sexual problem.

These are examples of this type of attacking dialogue:

"I keep doing different kinds of things like wearing sexy negligees, and you are still not turned on and getting an erection. I am sick of trying to give you an erection!" or, "I try this position and that position during intercourse and stimulate your clitoris with my hand until it is about ready to fall off, but nothing seems to give you an orgasm. I guess you are just a frigid woman and there is nothing I can do to change that fact."

These are statements of people who started out with good intentions of trying to "help" their partners. They have invested a great deal of their own ego and self-esteem in their efforts. Their excessive need to please and to rescue or be responsible is met with failure and frustration, and so they place the blame back on the partner they started out trying to please.

The antidote for the codependency syndrome is to develop the cognitive attitude of "caring enough not to care." This paradoxical idea frees the other partner from performance anxiety and demand for performance. It takes the focus off the sexual goal of the moment. On the surface, this type of thinking sounds heartless, but it is just the opposite. It is essential that a couple learn the value of temporary selfishness so they can lose themselves to the sexual experience.

For most people, caring means doing something for the person they care about. In some cases, helpful action does need to be taken; but often, such action can create unforeseen problems. In the case of sexual codependency, this is always the case. If your partner is experiencing some type of sexual dysfunction, you have to care enough to let your partner fix his or her own problem, rather than taking responsibility for it yourself. By jumping in and taking that responsibility away from your partner, you rob your lover of their own power to admit to the problem and seek lasting solutions.

Caring enough not to be codependent on the person you love frees you and your partner from performance anxiety and the demand for sexual goals. So often, when someone cares too much, the partner with the trouble feels a tremendous pressure to perform, to the degree that he or she may become inhibited and soon begin resisting any sexual involvement.

Spectatoring

When most people think of spectatoring as a sexual experience, they think of the sexual fetish of voyeurism, where someone derives sexual pleasure by spying on others involved in intimate sexual behaviors.

If we're going have a good sexual experience, we must be able to let ourselves be vulnerable. We need to be free of all distracting thoughts and lose ourselves in the moment. Sometimes, however, we worry about our sexual ability or our attractiveness, remaining outside the experience mentally, monitoring our emotions and watching the other person's as well. This behavior is known as spectatoring. Spectatoring has nothing to do with sexual pleasure; it's a source of sexual anxiety.

In spectatoring, one part of us is watching how we are responding sexually, another part is watching our partner, and still another part is watching how we are interacting. We may have an entire gallery of fragmentary selves watching the sexual event—with none of them actually participating.

The spectatoring person is in their head, barely making contact with their body. Naturally, their sexual feelings will become dulled. They are so busy watching and thinking that they forget the experience. It should be no surprise that they may not be able to let go and respond fully to the feelings that their senses are receiving. Often, a man who is spectatoring will not be able to achieve or maintain an erection. Similarly, a spectatoring woman may have difficulty experiencing orgasm.

Spectators do not mentally stand outside of themselves for the purpose of sexual arousal, as is the case with voyeurs. Instead, they tend to be sexually insecure, with a poor body image, or simply may be the victims of sexual perfectionism. When someone is watching his own or his partner's sexual behavior, he is taking a judgmental stance. As a result, his freedom and ability to be vulnerable and uninhibited are highly limited, to say the least.

With all this sexual spectatoring and judging going on during the sexual experience, it's easy to understand how this creates so much sexual performance anxiety. It reminds me of the Winter Olympics, when the figure skaters do their routines and the judges hold up cards with numbers rating the skaters' performances. I am sure that would create a lot of anxiety in the skater, especially if they made a mistake. That same process of judging is going on in a person's head as they are making love to their partner. Some women will only be involved sexually if they can turn all the lights off and make love in the dark. This way, they won't be physically judged because the spectator is blinded by the darkness.

Sometimes spectatoring serves as an escape mentally from the sexual experience. A person may use spectatoring as a defense mechanism in an uncomfortable situation. I find this to be the case with many women who have difficulty saying no to their partner's sexual advances. They give their bodies, but their minds are on something else—perhaps the shopping list. Why do they get involved in the first place, you might ask? There may be many reasons, but the one I hear the most often is that it is easier in the moment to give in than it is to refuse and then have to deal with repercussions. This may seem a satisfactory solution on a short-term basis, but the long-term consequences are incredibly destructive, both to the woman's sexuality and to the couple's relationship.

A man may use the same spectatoring technique for a different reason when he is experiencing premature ejaculation. He tries to remove himself from the sexual experience mentally so that he can control the degree of stimulation he is receiving, and therefore postpone ejaculation. The idea of removing yourself from the sexual experience is ridiculous, and isn't at all effective in treating premature ejaculation.

The antidote for spectatoring is to find the psychological issues that are causing the person to avoid fully participating sexually. What is the person avoiding through sexual spectatoring? What is the payoff, or how is it serving them in some way? Once these issues have been resolved (which will probably require psychotherapy), they can refocus their attention. For those who become sexual spectators only occasionally, the awareness experience described in Chapter Seven may be helpful.

Perfectionists who become spectators sexually need to readjust their attitude and expectations so that they are more in line with reality. They must realize that there is no perfect body and no perfect sexual experience. As the famous family therapist Virginia Satir wrote in her book, *Peoplemaking*, "Whenever you look for perfection you always find imperfection."(1) Perfection doesn't exist with humans. We are not machines or computer-enhanced images.

Every sexual experience is unique and special unto itself. The perfectionist tends to set up one real or imagined sexual experience as the ideal against which all others are compared. Disappointment is inevitable. Males who frequently watch pornography on the Internet are setting themselves up for the same kind of disappointment because they start to believe that the sex they watch on their computer is real; the lines between sexual fantasy and reality get blurred. They expect their real-life lovers to be like the women they watch on their computer where there is no emotional involvement. They may not know how to have sex with a real woman and may find it intimidating because the real deal requires them to be emotionally vulnerable—something that pornography doesn't ask of them.

Perfectionism is equally deadly when it relates to one's body image and sexual self-esteem and self-confidence. So often, I hear people complain that they are too small, too big, too skinny, or too fat. They are never satisfied with how their bodies look. They always point out some imperfection, whether it is a stretch mark here or a tiny scar there. As an associate of mine, Sheilah Fish, says, "They focus on the hole instead of the doughnut."

They are missing the big picture. When we compare our physical selves to images in television advertisements, the Internet, and all the other visual sources in the media, we guarantee ourselves an experience of inadequacy. Occasionally, it helps to remind ourselves—particularly the perfectionist in us—that those images in magazines are well doctored by sophisticated computer techniques that can completely alter the way women and men look. These techniques can take parts from different images and make a composite picture of a woman or man. In other cases, the image is completely computer generated. None of this has to do with the reality of what humans look like. Again, it is all fantasy.

It is difficult, especially for younger people, to realize that there is no such thing as perfection when it comes to bodies. Our daily lives are so saturated, via television, the Internet, and magazine advertising, with images of the ideal male and female physique, that we lose touch with reality. The challenge is to constantly remind ourselves that the media is full of unrealistic images, and buying the products they sell won't help us achieve the look they are promoting.

The point is to enjoy what assets you have and accept yourself exactly the way you are. Tell that perfectionist spectator to get lost because it is getting in the way of you enjoying yourself sexually, and in a bigger way, loving yourself fully.

Communication Breakdowns That Create Sexual Anxiety and Block Sexual Pleasure

Most couples find intimate verbal communication difficult. Talking specifically about sex is harder still. This, despite the fact that discussions about sex on television have become increasingly candid, with a plethora of shows on cable television describing the perfect orgasm and advising how to have great sex. On TV, we are constantly exposed to ads for erectile dysfunction medications showing happy, loving couples. All of this media bombardment on the masses has the effect of a "tabloid" approach to sex, which often creates more imaginary standards on how a couple should be in their sexual life.

The message that many of us get is that if we aren't having terrific sex all the time, then our relationship is in trouble, or we aren't part of a well-matched couple. Just as there are not perfect bodies, there is no perfect sexual relationship. When someone on television or in a magazine article or book says there is no excuse for not having great sex, it makes it harder than ever for a couple to admit that they have a problem. It is easier for them to pretend they are like everyone else—that is, like all the other people who are presumably having fantastic sex and who communicate well.

But when such a couple cannot talk intimately, they tend to make assumptions about what their partner wants sexually. Such assumptions create problems because neither person ends up receiving or giving what they really want.

Interacting sexually based on assumptions creates anxiety because without knowledge, fear is created. All the concerns about performance come into play. This fear and worry inhibit sexual pleasure from occurring.

Such assumptions may be based on what was true in the beginning of their relationship, but without continuing intimate communication, these assumptions have no way of being updated to fit both partners' changing attitudes and feelings. Since sexual preferences can change, it is important to regularly check out your assumptions about what your partner likes. Even long-standing couples can discover that they were incorrect in their outdated assumptions.

Sometimes I hear this type of communication between couples in therapy:

> "You mean you really like oral sex?"
> "Yes, I do."
> "You're kidding. I thought you hated it."
> "I did, but that was five years ago. I like it now."

I commonly ask the couples I see who come into my office, "Are you able to ask your partner to give you pleasure in specific ways?" My goal is to determine the level of sexual communication present in the relationship. For the majority of couples in sex therapy, the answer to this question is no.

A couple's inability to communicate sets them up for routine, predictable sex. Their effectiveness at giving each other pleasure is greatly reduced. They tend to make love as if they are in a fog, automatically going through the same motions over and over, with little thought about exactly what they are doing.

For people unable to communicate sexually, the thought of straying from the beaten track and asking for something different from their partner can be extremely threatening. Often, the partner who desires a certain kind of sexual contact is afraid that the other partner will think of them as being selfish, demanding, or even perverse.

The way to break through this fear is to make it clear to your partner that just because you ask for something does not mean that you require compliance. You are simply offering information about what feels good to you, and your partner can use this information in whatever way he or she feels comfortable. If you do go about your sexual communication with the attitude that you expect to get everything you ask for, then you are indeed being selfish and aggressive. If this is your expectation of sex, then it is probably best that you live alone.

On the other hand, not expressing your desires leaves your sexual experience a mystery to your partner. This will set them up for a sense of frustration, failure, and a whole lot of anxiety because your partner doesn't know how to give you what you want. As we saw in Chapter Six, many women are afraid to express their sexual desires verbally because they don't want to hurt their partner's feelings. They are afraid they will make their partner feel inadequate at his assumed job of being the all-knowing sex expert.

Sometimes, a woman expresses her sexual desires verbally, but feels she has been rejected. Asking for what you want sexually puts you in a psychologically vulnerable situation, so it seems less stressful and safer simply not to be assertive. Many men also fall into this way of thinking. The problem with this nonassertive, self-protective approach is that it stunts the growth and activity in a sexual relationship. You may be protecting yourself from the emotional pain of perceived rejection, but at the same time, you are cheating yourself out of the possibility of a fulfilling sexual life.

Our fears of talking about sex tend to be strongest while we are in the midst of sexual interaction. To overcome these fears, it is important to understand the emotional costs in the long run if these fears are left unresolved. Take the example of the woman who doesn't want to threaten her partner or make him feel inadequate as a lover. After a period of time of not getting her sexual needs fulfilled, she will probably lose interest in her partner. Her partner will then take her sexual apathy very personally, since he will not understand the reasons for her lack of interest. By protecting him from the relatively minor discomfort that communicating her needs might have provoked, she has set up a situation in which he will be far more deeply hurt in the long run because of her lack of sexual interest.

Many women have told me in therapy that they gave their partner specific verbal instructions as to what gives them sexual pleasure, but with poor results. A woman might say, "I told him to touch my clitoris gently, not as if he were polishing a car, but he keeps doing it the same way. What is the point of communicating? He just ignores me."

We can all understand this woman's frustration, but I would advise her to keep trying to communicate with him. She does need to stop participating sexually if her partner does not respect her desires or does not tell her honestly when he doesn't want to do what she requests, or ignores her.

Summary

In establishing a long-term pleasurable relationship, it is essential to open yourself to communicate with your sexual partner. Frank, open talk is the vehicle by which we get the information necessary to give our lovers pleasure throughout the relationship. Because this information changes all the time, there needs to be a constant updating in order to stay current with our partner's changing desires and physical needs. It is the continual exchange of information that keeps a couple from falling into a predictable sexual routine.

I don't mean to suggest that you and your partner need to forcibly maintain a constant discussion of your sexual wants and desires. My point is just that direct and clear verbal communication is necessary, especially at the beginning of a relationship when you know so little about each other. But after a while, a few comments here and there may be all that is required: "Oh, that feels great!" or "A little harder, please." Just like when you are telling someone how to scratch your back and get at the point where you just can't reach, but when they do, it feels so good.

Small directional cues will usually suffice. If you become too verbally focused, then you will be thinking so much that you may forget to actually experience the physical pleasure. In addition, there are nonverbal ways of communicating. Good lovers can read the nonverbal cues of their partners in order to get information as to how their partner is experiencing certain physical stimulation. Nonverbal signals can include heart rate, breathing rate, muscular tension, facial expressions, and sounds such as moans and groans. Also, moving your partner's hands in a directive way can give indications about what you want.

If there is a single principle that holds true throughout this discussion, it is that where long-term relationships are concerned, there's a good reason that sexual intercourse is described as making love. Without caring and respect for our self and our partner, there is little chance of enjoying any depth of sexual intimacy. Both partners need to be able to lose themselves to each other. This level of caring and respect requires self-understanding, self-responsibility, and a genuine interest in our partner's, as well as our own, human needs, human weaknesses, and human strengths. When all this comes together in the playful, pleasure-oriented way that our sexuality offers, few activities are more fulfilling.

Works Cited

1. Satir, Virginia. *The New Peoplemaking*. Palo Alto, CA: Science and Behavior Books, 1988.

13

Taking Your Passion and Making It Happen

Thus far, we have discussed many ideas about achieving fulfilling sexual relationships. To a large extent, we've explored them out of context; that is, as isolated events in a person's life. In this chapter, we'll be taking a slightly different approach, showing how we put all these ideas together by outlining a couple's sex therapy program.

This is a way to take all the cognitive concepts discussed in previous chapters and illustrate how they become integrated behaviorally. Sexual interaction isn't just about theoretical concepts, but behavior as well. Sex therapy is a good practical example of the cognitive/behavioral approach to psychological therapy.

Rather than being intended for self-help, I offer this information for couples who want to enrich an already good sexual relationship and for couples who are experiencing problems and want a mental picture of what would be involved if they sought the help of a qualified sex therapist.

Dr. Tom Lowry, MD, taught the basic format of this material to me, along with his wife, Thea Lowry, MA, who worked with Masters and Johnson in their clinic in St. Louis, Missouri, during the early 1970s. I have altered certain parts to make the program more effective for my patients. Some therapists call the techniques of this program sensate focus exercises. I see them as more than that. What I am trying to do essentially is to help a sexually dysfunctional couple restructure their sexual relationship into a mutually fulfilling experience. It is this restructuring process that I call sex therapy.

Most couples who come to me for help seem to have a set routine in the way they make love. While these routines are not necessarily bad, their predictability hardly fosters excitement. When couples experience real difficulties, the routines they established are usually not just lackluster, but actually antierotic, inhibiting sexual pleasure. For them, it is imperative that they restructure the ways in which they are sexually involved. Otherwise, the future of their marriage may be at risk.

A couple can go about restructuring their sexual relationship in a step-by-step progression, moving on to the next step only when they have successfully completed the one they are on. Success occurs at the point at which they have both become comfortable and have had pleasure doing the prescribed exercises.

The couple should have no goals while going through the therapeutic process. While the therapist does have goals in mind, the couple's responsibility is simply to experience pleasure. People entering therapy tend to be very goal oriented. They are so focused on their problem that this focus itself becomes an obstacle. They have worked and worked on their own to improve their sexual relationship, but to no avail. By the time they seek therapy, they are very frustrated, and it is difficult for them to let go of their goals.

It is important for a couple experiencing difficulties to understand that no one is to blame for their problems. All blaming must cease. Both people in a relationship contribute to every aspect of that relationship, the good and the bad. It may be hard for each one to see his or her contribution to the problem, but until blaming stops, it is almost impossible to establish an atmosphere of emotional comfort and vulnerability. The absence of blame allows each person to make changes in his or her behavior without having past mistakes brought up again. As Dr. Lowry used to say during my training, "It took both of you to get off track, so it's going to take both of you to get back on."

Another prerequisite for participating in this process is that the couple be in relatively good emotional shape. Couples at war are not good candidates for sex therapy. If one of the partners has recently had an affair that the other partner has discovered, they are likewise poor candidates. These couples will probably get the best results if they seek out marriage therapy first. Two people have to be lovers outside the bedroom before they can be good lovers in the bedroom. Emotional well-being is the foundation from which sex therapy proceeds. Many times, couples seeking sex therapy need to work on their communication skills and conflict resolution skills through general marriage therapy before they are ready to improve their sexual relationship.

I will describe the process using an example couple, John and Jane, speaking as though they were in my office going through the therapy process. Assuming that John and Jane have met the above criteria and are good sex therapy candidates, we are ready to start the program. In the example that follows, the couple determined through mutual consent that Jane would take the initiative and that she would take responsibility for details such as preparing the atmosphere in the bedroom. While it doesn't matter which partner starts, there will usually be one or the other who will volunteer. Very often, this turns out to be the person who sought help from the therapist and made the first appointment.

Step One

Jane, sometime in the next few days, I would like you to initiate the following exercise with John. And John, if you are not interested at the time Jane initiates it, then say no to her request. If you are neutral about participating, then lend yourself to the experience and see what happens. It is important that both of you want to participate.

Jane, I would like you to create a setting that is inviting for you and John to be sexually involved with each other. Check the lighting. You don't want it to be too bright, so that you feel as if you are on an operating table, or too dark, so you can't see your partner's body. An aromatic candle would do the trick. In addition to the lighting, the temperature of the room is very important. It can't be too cold because then it might not be comfortable to remove your clothes. Along with the lighting and temperature, Jane, you might also want to attend to things that promote a feeling of romance and sensuality, such as soft background music, incense, or whatever works for you and John.

I want you to choose a time to be together when you won't be watching the clock. You are not in any hurry to go do something else because if you are thinking about the time, it will get in the way of enjoying the experience to its fullest. If you feel you are in hurry, it might be best not to start this exercise until you have more time.

Privacy is another important factor. If you and John are worried that one of your children will walk in on you, you're going to feel inhibited and it will limit your level of pleasure. If you need to put a lock on the bedroom door for comfort, then do so. You need to feel that you have some place that belongs just to the two of you, as a couple. There needs to be a psychological, as well as physical, boundary between a couple and their children. Otherwise, the couple's relationship will be lost in the identity of the family.

Assuming all the necessary criteria have been met, Jane, you are ready to begin. You and John are in a nice, comfortable setting, with no particular place to go or be other than with each other.

I want you both to be naked. Clothes only get in the way. In whatever position you both find comfortable, I want you, Jane, to touch John's body for your own pleasure and information. I don't want you to try to turn him on sexually or to give him an erection or an orgasm. I don't want you to think of him at all. I want you to pay attention to what you find pleasurable.

Now, when Jane is touching you for her own pleasure, John, I want you to agree to something. I want you to agree to communicate with Jane in a nonverbal way when you find her touch unpleasurable to you. Do this by gently moving her hand to another location on your body.

Jane, given that John has agreed to communicate to you if he is having a problem with your touching him, you can feel free from worrying about John. If he leaves your hand alone, everything is fine with him. So, back to touching John. I want you to touch him all over his body, from head to toe if you like. The only exception is that I want you to stay away from his genitals. For now, that area is off limits. Everywhere else is great.

Touch his face, his back, and chest all the way down to his feet. The only off-limits area for touching is his genitals. If you are using your hands to touch him, pretend the nerve endings in your fingers are plugged into an amplifier. I want you turn the volume up full blast. I want you to notice what feels soft, smooth, warm, hairy, hard—notice every detail and nuance. Fully concentrate on what you feel—not on what you think or perceive in your environment.

(I often refer patients to the awareness experience described earlier in this book in Chapter Seven. Its application can be invaluable for this exercise.)

I recognize that having someone tell you how to touch your husband may seem awkward. I expect that when you first start touching John, you may not feel comfortable. I hope you are comfortable, but if you are not, I understand. I realize also that this experience may seem clinical, unromantic, programmed, or not spontaneous, but that is okay. It is something new and different, and a certain amount of discomfort and doubt is normal. I want you to go through the awkward stage until you start to relax, and then continue as long as you like, just touching John for your own pleasure. Jane, you can touch John as long as you want and as long as is comfortable for John. When you are ready to, you can stop.

When Jane is done touching you, John, it is now your turn to touch her. While touching, refrain from talking. Use no verbal instructions or comments whatsoever. When people start verbalizing during a sexual experience, their mental focus tends to shift from what they are feeling to what they are thinking. This shift can inhibit them from fully experiencing the touching, both in the giving and receiving positions.

When Jane touches John for her pleasure or John touches Jane, the person being touched should be aware of what he or she is feeling. The individual should be open to the pleasure of this experience, while following the instructions to gently move the toucher's hand to a different location if something is not pleasurable.

John, now that it is your turn to touch Jane, follow the same touch procedure that Jane did, but with a few exceptions. Again, you are touching her for your own pleasure. You are not trying to arouse her or give her an orgasm. You have no goals, only the experience of the pleasure of the moment.

Jane, if John touches you in a place or in a way that is not pleasurable to you, then you will agree to move his hand to a more neutral place. So, John, since you do not have to worry about what you are doing to Jane, you can be uninhibited in your pleasure. You will not have distracting thoughts such as, "She is irritated with the way I touch her," or "She hates it when I touch her stomach lightly." You can assume that if Jane does not move your hand away, you are not doing anything that bothers her.

Touch her whole body, with the exception of her breasts and genitals. Avoid these areas. But touching her everywhere else is fine. Again, I want you to touch her as long as it is mutually comfortable.

When you have both touched each other in this way, stop. Go no further. This experience is not to lead to intercourse. You may be thinking, "What? No sex? I thought this was sex therapy!" I urge you to be patient if the process doesn't go as you might have fantasized it.

Many men object to what they call "touchy-feely" experiences of this sort. They say it is just an excuse used by women who feel uncomfortable, to put off sex. Until the man is willing to look beyond this and give the exercises a chance, the therapy cannot proceed.

After this experience has been completed once, I ask the couple to do it one more time. Everything should be repeated exactly the same, except that whoever initiated the first experience will be the one to be touched first this time. The one who received first in the initial experience will be the initiator in the second.

Issues in Step One

Sometimes, when a couple returns after this exercise, one of them says, "Well, nothing happened. I didn't feel anything." Invariably, we find that the person who says this was expecting some big turn-on or a raving sexual experience. That is not the point of this exercise. The only purpose is to provide an opportunity for both participants to experience and become aware of all the more subtle sensations of their sexuality, to become sensual people. This is the quality that is missing in so many long-term relationships. It is all the little sensations that create so much pleasure. When a person becomes so goal oriented that all they think about is achieving a big turn-on or having intercourse and subsequent orgasm, that person is going to miss all the little sensations involved. As a result, the degree of sexual pleasure actually enjoyed is greatly reduced.

In this experience, a couple has the opportunity to go back to their adolescence, back to a time when all they could do was to touch or hold hands. Holding hands can be a very erotic experience if one pays attention to all the little, pleasurable sensations. By giving up the goal of intercourse and orgasm during the touching experience, they are forced to keep their mental focus in the present. They can't go anywhere else mentally if they stay within the bounds of the therapy. What many couples discover is that this experience is extremely sexual, even though intercourse and orgasm are not part of the experience.

The Removal of Goals

For the man who is experiencing some type of sexual dysfunction, the removal of the goal of intercourse is a great relief. For example, if he is having problems with erections or premature ejaculation, he will feel relieved that he won't have to perform. His anxiety level will drop dramatically. As a result of his reduction of anxiety, he will be able to relax and enjoy much more of the sexual pleasure he is experiencing. With the use of erectile dysfunction medication, the same reduction of anxiety can occur, allowing the male to relax, which enables him to focus on the pleasure of the moment; as a result, he can achieve an erection. During the exercise, he is instructed to just enjoy the fact that he has an erection, but not do anything with it.

Once relaxation occurs, the sexual dysfunction he was experiencing should decrease. Right away, the therapy is structured to break the typical, problematic goal-oriented loop that is associated with most sexual dysfunctions. It is easy to tell someone with sexual dysfunctions to relax and not worry about the problem, but without a safe structure and strict guidelines to follow, the anxiety will remain.

The outcome of a couple's experience with this exercise tells the therapist as well as the couple a great deal about the degree of intimacy that exists in the relationship. If one or possibly both of the partners has a lot of repressed anger, they will probably report after their experience of touching each other that they didn't feel much when being touched. It is hard to be close to someone you are angry with, even if your anger is repressed or unconscious. Instead of feeling pleasure, the individual experiences being uncomfortable or irritated because touching makes them aware of their resentments. Since they don't wish to acknowledge the resentments, they repress them and resist the touching experience by numbing their senses.

It becomes obvious to a couple that they are avoiding each other if they somehow are not creating any time to participate in the sex therapy assignments. Usually, when this happens, the therapy process changes focus from sexual intimacy to building greater communication and emotional intimacy.

Vulnerability and Control Issues

Another issue this exercise tends to bring to the surface is the couple's ability to be vulnerable within a sexual context. This becomes evident in the reaction of the partner, when he or she is on the receiving end of the touching experience. The person on the receiving end is in a vulnerable position; they are not in control, except by moving the partner's hand if they are uncomfortable with how they are being touched. That partner is in the position of being a part of a sexual experience without being able to set its tempo, style, or direction. For people who are uncomfortable with being vulnerable in this way, the exercise can be very difficult. They like to be in control of what occurs in a sexual context. They will have trouble relaxing and keeping themselves from telling their partner how to touch them.

The hope is that with repeated experience, the individual with vulnerability issues will be able to let go of control and develop trust with their partner and be able to relax.

Another indication of difficulty with being physically vulnerable is when a person responds by being ticklish. Being ticklish to tactile stimulation is a way of guarding yourself from what you may perceive as an intrusion into your personal space. If someone comes up behind you silently and gives you a surprise tickle, you jump and your body tenses. It was a surprise intrusion, and you suddenly felt that you had to guard your body. Ticklishness is a learned response and can be overcome. Often, people claim they are ticklish because they are unusually sensitive; while this may be partly true, the primary cause of ticklishness is fear of vulnerability. It is a symptom, rather than a problem in itself.

Beneficial Selfishness

Probably the greatest benefit of this touching exercise is discovering that you can touch your partner for your own pleasure. This idea is very foreign to many people because it implies selfishness, which has a very negative connotation in our culture. As Dr. Helen Singer Kaplan states in her book, *The New Sex Therapy*, "It is often essential to teach the couple the value of temporary selfishness so that they can lose themselves to the sexual experience."(1) She also says, "To function well sexually, the individual(s) must be able to abandon themselves to the erotic experience."(2)

Being selfish usually implies that you do what you want, regardless of other people's wishes; this is not what I am recommending when I instruct couples to touch for their own pleasure. I want them to focus on their own pleasure, but not at the expense of their partner's pleasure and sexual experience. This is why the instructions to the receiving partner are to move the hand of the partner if anything is uncomfortable. This is important because it gives the touching partner freedom from the worry of pleasing the receiver and lets the giver have the opportunity to lose him- or herself to the sexual experience.

People who have an excessive need to please their partners also have difficulty with this exercise. To sexually interact for their own pleasure can put them into an emotional bind, allowing them to begin to come to terms with their need to give and to begin accepting pleasure more openly.

Communicating Trust

Another psychological issue raised by this sexual experience is trusting that your partner will communicate their sexual discomforts. By experiencing the other partner moving your hand to other locations during the sexual exercise, you can learn that your partner can take care of him- or herself. This relieves the anxiety caused by trying to be responsible for your partner's sexual experience.

Through this exercise, the couple builds a foundation of trust, allowing both partners to abandon themselves to their own sexual pleasure. This exercise reinforces the idea that each partner will take responsibility for his or her own sexuality, freeing both of them to relax and become vulnerable.

Time for Intimacy

Many couples' sexual and/or emotional difficulties stem from the fact that they do not allow time for intimacy in their daily lives. Often, the demands of today's lifestyles—two careers, two children, and complex social involvements—don't leave much time, even for a couple who aren't experiencing other difficulties. But when problems are present, the couple can be so busy that they don't have much time for each other. They try to maintain a status quo and avoid any intense emotional confrontation. At some level, they may know that they don't have the skills to handle too much intimate contact.

This exercise confronts the problem of time head on. It forces the couple to look at where they place their time, how they choose to budget it, and where their priorities lie in terms of the importance they place on time alone together. Just creating intimate time together to participate in this exercise may be difficult. They may come back to the next therapy session with all sorts of excuses as to why they couldn't find time to do the home experiences. They may be afraid to do the exercises, but more often I find that they have created routines that simply allow no time for intimacy.

At this point where the couple realize they have literally scheduled sexuality and intimacy out of their lives, they have a choice to either continue in that way or give their sexuality an opportunity to flourish. Assuming that they choose the latter, they make a date to spend some intimate time together. Given their lifestyles, they are reminded that this kind of time is not going to appear magically. They have to create it, even if it means sitting down with their calendars and blocking in time for their relationship.

If there are underlying unresolved emotions and issues in their relationship, these may have to be resolved before this exercise is going to be helpful to them.

The Erogenous Body

Another concept this exercise brings into play is that the whole body is an erogenous zone. By making the breasts and genitals (usually the main targets of sexual stimulation) off limits, they turn their sensual attention to all the other parts of their bodies. The couple learns that they can derive pleasure from stimulation that doesn't include genital arousal. In this way, they begin to experience the difference between sensual and sexual stimulation.

When a couple's sexuality is goal oriented—that is, oriented toward orgasm and little, if anything, in between, this exercise holds quite a few surprises for them. The man may get upset and confused about why his efforts do not lead to intercourse. As often as not, however, after two or three touching experiences, they begin to forget about their sexual goals, focusing instead on the pleasure of the moment and learning to relax and have fun with sex. Besides learning the pleasure of the moment, they learn new information about their own bodies, as well as their partner's. They learn which areas of their bodies are sensitive and which are not.

Follow the Rules

Occasionally, after a couple comes back to therapy after their first week of doing that first step of touching, they act a little sheepish and giggle. I ask them what's up. They respond with, "Well we didn't follow the rules you gave in the assignment." I ask, "What do you mean, you didn't follow the rules?" "Well, we started doing the touching as you prescribed, and all of sudden I started getting an erection. I couldn't believe it! So I had to use it and have intercourse, even though you said no intercourse." "That's true, but what happened once you started having intercourse?" "I lost my erection." "I know; see what happens when you don't follow doctor's orders? Well, the good news is you can do the exercise again, but this time, follow the rules. I want you to have the attitude that if you get an erection, no big deal, there are many more where that came from, so no need to panic."

Step Two

In the next step of the therapy, Jane, you are to be the initiator as before, creating a sensual environment. The major difference is that this time when you are touching John's body, you can include his genitals. The idea of touching for your own pleasure still applies. Also, there is still no goal to this experience, even though you may be touching his penis. If he gets an erection, fine, but if he doesn't, that is also fine, because that is not the point of the experience. If he ejaculates while you are stimulating him, that is nice for him, but it is not the point of this step in the therapy process.

Another change I would like to make is that when Jane is touching you, John, in addition to moving her hand away from what is not pleasurable, I want you to move her hand in a way that will show her what would be more pleasurable to you. This is a way to show Jane not only what is uncomfortable, but also what gives you the most pleasure. This part of the exercise carries the assumption that Jane finds what you want her to do with her hands pleasurable and comfortable as well. This form of communication and education is essential in learning to be more effective lovers.

When you have touched him for as long as you want, Jane, it is John's turn to touch you, in the same way with all the same instructions in mind. Just because I have said that you can touch her breasts and genitals, John, I don't want you to focus on these areas. Don't forget, the rest of her body has nerve endings, too! Again, this exercise is for your own pleasure; you are not trying to achieve any goal or meet any expectation. Just because you can touch Jane's genitals doesn't mean that you should try to give her an orgasm. Touch her genitals because it gives you pleasure. If she happens to have an orgasm, that's nice for her, but that is not the goal. As with the first part of step two, Jane, I want you to move John's hands in a manner that shows what is most pleasurable to you.

This experience is not to include intercourse. This limitation is very important and often you may find it difficult to adhere to, but it is the key to the process. Once John is done touching you, Jane, then the experience is complete. If you both want to talk over what the experience was like for you, that is fine, but only after the actual touching is completed for both of you.

On a separate occasion, John is to be the initiator.

One recommendation I make at this stage of the therapy process is the use of skin lubricant. I suggest its use only in the genital areas. Given the high concentration of nerve endings there, lubrication will cut down on irritating friction. Skin rubbing on skin in a highly sensitive nerve area is not usually pleasurable. The addition of lubrication will add to the sensuality of the experience. A lubricant I usually recommend is Unscented Albolene Moisturizing Cleanser. It melts on contact with the skin to the consistency of natural sexual lubricant, but is longer lasting. It is intended as a makeup remover and skin moisturizer, so when you go to the drugstore to buy some, you won't feel embarrassed because only you know what you will use it for.

Issues in Step Two

This second step helps the partners provide each other with a map to the territory. By directing their partner as to what gives them pleasure, John and Jane take full responsibility for their own sexuality. John shows Jane how he likes his penis stimulated. The penis is similar to the clitoris and has various responses to different forms of stimulation. Some areas of the penis are more sensitive than others, and, of course, this varies from one person to another. Some men like their penis stroked slowly, others fast, or both. Once again, it varies from man to man or even from day to day with the same man. The point of all this is that specific communication is required, so that Jane will not be just traveling around, lost in sexual territory without a map, an exercise that frustrates both partners.

The communication of specific sexual desires and stimulation is important for both partners, of course. Often, it seems the men I see in therapy have very limited knowledge about how to stimulate their partner's clitoris. Some men aren't even aware of its location.

As with the penis, the clitoris requires different types of stimulation, varying greatly from woman to woman. Some women prefer one side of their clitoris to the other, where others like circling stimulation around the organ. The same woman may want to be stimulated one way in one situation and another way the next time they make love. So, it is important for a woman to communicate to her lover how she wants to be stimulated each time. Just assuming that your partner knows what to do is setting yourself up for frustration.

Ideally, this communication about how she would like to have her genitals stimulated should be given nonverbally, though sometimes a few words may need to be said. Remember, however, that long discourses get in the way of the experience.

The best way for a woman to show a man how she would like her clitoris to be stimulated is for her to place her hand on his and lead him. This is better than telling him verbally, because she is receiving stimulation from him at the same time that she is teaching him. A major issue about sexual responsibility for the man is addressed at this point. This occurs when his partner becomes more assertive about her specific sexual needs.

Men who are not entirely secure about their sexual confidence and self-esteem may feel threatened and uncomfortable with being instructed by their lover. They may perceive this instruction as a put-down of their sexual ability, and they can become resistant to doing what their partner asks. Through the therapy process, the man begins to understand that when his partner gives him information about what pleasures her, it enables him to be a more effective lover. Any man doing this exercise should be reminded beforehand that there is no way that he could have known this very specific kind of information without his partner communicating it to him. Regardless of his experience as a lover, only her instructions can tell him what works for her.

Sex Does Not Equal Intercourse

The next issue addressed at this part of the therapy is being sexual without intercourse. In the first step of therapy, we are exploring sensuality or touching for the sake of pleasure. Here, we are adding stimulation of the genitals to the sensual experience. For many couples who are experiencing sexual dysfunctions or sexual boredom, this step can be difficult. They are used to feeling that once they become sexually aroused, they must immediately commence with intercourse. This step in the therapy blocks that goal-oriented mentality and forces the couple to focus on the pleasure of the moment. It is no accident that many couples compare this experience to make-out sessions they had when they were in high school.

The ability to enjoy sex without having intercourse gives the couple variety and flexibility in their shared sexuality. They can break out of the meat-and-potatoes style of lovemaking. Men who experience problems with premature ejaculation or erection difficulty give a sigh of relief when they are told not to engage in intercourse. This is especially true for a man who is anxious about controlling his ejaculation. The pressure is lifted from him, and he can be sexually involved with his partner—perhaps for the first time. If he does ejaculate before his partner has experienced orgasm, he doesn't have to feel inadequate. He can use other means—his hands or mouth—to stimulate his partner. Added to that, he's almost home in correcting his dysfunction.

For women who are preorgasmic, this stage of the therapy is especially significant. It is critical for a woman to be able to communicate to her lover the specific forms of sexual stimulation she needs. This juncture of the process also validates and supports the realization that it is perfectly fine to be orgasmic without intercourse. For women who feel inadequate if they aren't orgasmic while receiving stimulation through intercourse, only this part of the therapy relieves them of that anxiety.

Learning to Receive Pleasure

Like the first stage of the process, the second stage puts partners in positions that are emotionally and physically vulnerable. Unlike the first stage, this vulnerability now comes from allowing the partner to touch the most intimate parts of the body. The partner who is being touched is forced to indulge him- or herself in receiving a tremendous amount of intense sexual pleasure. That might sound like heaven to some people, but for others, this kind of vulnerability produces more anxiety than pleasure. This step in the process provides a safe setting for this type of person to better understand his or her fear of losing control. It lets both partners abandon themselves to sexual pleasure.

This is the point where more traditional psychotherapy techniques may be employed. The roots of a person's fear of sexual vulnerability may need to be examined and understood. Without this insight, their fears run their lives. Psychotherapy can lead them toward making choices that allow them to both enjoy their sexuality and feel safe, thus surrendering their need for control.

Step Three

After John and Jane have completed and enjoyed the first two steps, they are ready to move on to the third. In this exercise, we reintroduce the experience of intercourse. Jane is to initiate this only when she is ready to have intercourse with John. The recommended position when Jane is ready is called the female-astride position. John lies on his back, with Jane on top of him. During intercourse with Jane, John should take a passive role. That doesn't mean he should mentally check out. Rather, he can relax and enjoy receiving pleasure. In this case, passive simply means not trying to control the experience, unless John experiences some discomfort, in which case he needs to speak up about it.

With this step, Jane, I want you to be the initiator again, except this time, both of you are going to touch each other at the same time. It will be the same when John initiates the session.

Jane, you should be the one to orchestrate what happens while you and John are having intercourse. You control the rate of first penetration. Once John is inside, just sit there for a moment and let your vagina adjust to John's penis. After this pause, you are free to do whatever is comfortable or pleasurable for you. If you want to move slowly or if you want to move fast, it is up to you. As was the case with the other steps in the therapy, there is no goal in this step. If orgasms happen for either of you, that is great, but it is not the goal. If one of you doesn't experience an orgasm, there is no failure on anybody's part, as long as you are both feeling pleasure. This experience will end whenever one of you wants to stop. On another occasion, John, you are to initiate the whole experience, following the same procedure.

The Issues in Step Three

The issues with this step are related to the introduction of intercourse. It is important that Jane initiate intercourse during the pleasuring process because in most cases, the man initiates it, signaled only by his own arousal and his getting an erection. The problem with this is that although he may be ready, his partner may not be. Most men can't recognize when a woman is ready to have intercourse, unless she provides him with very specific signals such as pulling him to her in a way that makes it very clear that this is what she wants. The woman often consents to intercourse when she isn't ready, just because she feels inadequate at not being as aroused as her partner.

By agreeing to have intercourse when she is not sufficiently lubricated and aroused, the woman limits the level of sexual pleasure she can experience. It is equivalent to a man trying to have intercourse without an erection—not too much fun! If this pattern of behavior continues on a long-term basis, it may turn her off to intercourse entirely—all without her partner knowing what is happening. As far as he knows, she is enjoying what is occurring, and he continues to initiate whenever he is ready. A more experienced man might know better, but not unless he had either studied female sexuality or been instructed by a woman. After penetration, it is important for the woman to let her vagina adjust to the penis. As discussed in Chapter Four on anatomy, the vagina is relatively closed prior to stimulation. It needs time to relax, expand, and lubricate. Otherwise, the woman might experience uncomfortable friction, which could lead to vaginismus, which was discussed in Chapter Eleven.

Allowing the Woman to Be in Control

With the woman on top in this exercise and the man relatively passive, the woman has the opportunity to assert herself. With the more common man-on-top missionary position, she is flattened under his weight. He orchestrates the whole experience. He sets the speed and tempo and depth of penetration. He is in control of the experience because she is not in a position to do much about it.

When the woman is on top, she has a chance to express herself. She can do whatever is pleasurable for her. Alexandra Penny states in her book, *How to Make Love to a Man*, "Some women say that they are reluctant to suggest this position because they feel they might appear overly aggressive. On the contrary, for many men this is the most erotic way to make love."(3) In this position, she is able to give herself or her partner additional manual stimulation, or her partner can give either or both of them stimulation from below. This could definitely increase pleasure over just having intercourse, something that can be especially important for a woman who doesn't experience orgasms through intercourse alone and would like to experience orgasms while having intercourse with her partner.

By remaining passive, the man learns to relinquish control and allow himself to be vulnerable. For some men, this is no problem, but for others, losing control can be threatening. In the latter case, the man can learn to lie back and receive the pleasure he is experiencing during this step in the therapy process. If he has trouble participating at this point, then the therapist can help him explore the fears he may be experiencing. This therapy might include traditional insight therapy with a behavioral process of confrontation, taking what is learned from the verbal part of the therapy and applying it to actual behavioral changes.

As an aside, the female-astride position is also very useful when the man is working on his ejaculation control. It allows him to control the level of stimulation because he can signal to his partner to pull off when he is coming close to ejaculating. Also, he has gravity on his side. When he is on top, he has to tighten up to support his body. In the female-astride position, this is not the case. His entire body can be at rest, except for his erect penis. This ability to physically relax is an essential component in controlling the timing of his ejaculation.

Step Four

By this point in the therapeutic process, John and Jane have integrated some of the major concepts of this book. They have broken and changed whatever sexual patterns that may have trapped them in an unsatisfactory sexual relationship.

The last step for you, John and Jane, is to do whatever you are comfortable doing, in whatever order or sequence you choose, and for however long. The purpose of the therapy is not to set up another rigid pattern. The idea is to be creative and free, to mix all the steps you have learned—for example, a little general body touching, some missionary-style intercourse, a little genital touching, and then back to intercourse, using a different position of your choosing.

Now that the level of pleasure has been increased, I might suggest that the partners talk to one another a little more during the sexual experience. For some, this can be just as exciting as touch.

The point is to try not to follow the same old pattern. Instead of playing the same five notes over and over in the same order, you now have a full range of notes and chords, and the combinations are endless. Instead of playing a half-hearted duet, you're now able to enjoy a full orchestra.

This might sound somewhat corny, but I think I have figured out where the metaphor of fireworks comes from, as applied to sex. A good fireworks show is just one beautiful explosion after another. When they have no rigid pattern, the couple has the freedom to be inventive and spontaneous. Their sexual experience becomes one fantastic pleasuring activity after another. The trick is to make it last. Like rich food, you can only have so much of it, but your mind still wants more. This is the way I hope you view your own sexual relationship.

Conclusion

Once the couple has mastered the mechanics of sex—the technique—the next order of business is to come back to the fundamental question of feelings. How do you feel about your partner? How do you feel about yourself? Do you like what you are doing? These are much tougher questions than questions of technique because they are about how we experience life, not just how we do sexual things.

"Ours is a culture that makes figuring out how to be physically sexual so complicated that many people never get to the question of how they feel about it," says John Gagnon in his book, *Human Sexuality*.(4) The key to long-term sexual fulfillment in a relationship is not usually what physical position a couple uses or what sexual technique they employ, but rather what their feelings or emotions are toward each other. The way a couple interacts physically is important, but it plays a secondary role to their emotional interactions. Every therapist has known at least one divorcing couple who said, "Oh, the sex was fine, but that's all we had between us. It wasn't enough." Of course, there many more couples who don't have much of a sex life due to the fact that they aren't emotionally intimate.

When they talk about their sex lives, most couples use the word love to describe how they feel. However, being emotionally involved or in love with a long-term partner doesn't mean that you will only experience warm, affectionate feelings. A committed relationship involves all the emotions of the human experience. Anger and related emotions are very important to the quality and intensity of a couple's sexual experience.

The repression, denial, or avoidance of anger is a sure ticket to the sexual doldrums. With so many couples, the primary reason they have turned from lovers into roommates is that they have repressed resentments and hurts in their relationship. When this happens, it takes a lot more than changing rooms to go from being roommates back to being lovers.

The key for couples who want to have more than just sex in their life is to find constructive ways to communicate—both the easy and the difficult emotions. Open communication may not be the only component in a good sex life, but it's way ahead of whatever is in second place.

I hope now you know what the title of this book, The Good Sex Bible means in real life. My concern is that the average person doesn't have a clue as to what I am talking about. With so many boys learning about sex from what they see in the form of pornography on the Internet, how will this play out in their interpersonal lives when they are older and married? How is this pornographic approach going to impact their lovers? What kinds of unrealistic expectations will this form of sexual learning set them up for in their sex lives? Now that you have finished this book, I hope this material will act as an antidote to the media's pornographic version of sexuality, which seems to be devoid of real sexual intimacy—as opposed to just sex—because the latter is so boring and loveless.

I don't want to end this book on a negative note. When a couple takes emotional intimacy and combines it with a sensual, flowing, pleasurable sexual interaction, they create a relationship that will never be boring, mechanical, and ultimately unfulfilling. My goal in writing The Good Sex Bible was to explain and illustrate this type of sexual relationship. Please enjoy.

Aloha,
Dan Beaver
Walnut Creek, California

Works Cited

1. Singer Kaplan, Helen, MD, PhD. *The New Sex Therapy.* New York: Taylor and Francis Group, 1974.
2. Singer Kaplan, Helen, MD, PhD. *The New Sex Therapy.* New York: Taylor and Francis Group, 1974.
3. Penney, Alexandra. *How to Make Love to a Man.* New York: Gramercy Books, 1981.
4. Gagnon, John. *Human Sexuality in Today's World.* Chicago: Scott Foresman & Co., 1977.

Acknowledgments

Many people contributed to the evolution of this book in its current form. For all their help and training, I wish to thank Thea Lowry-Snyder, MA, wherever her spirit may rest, and Tom Lo wry, MD. I also want to acknowledge the following people: my early co-therapists, Bonnie Darwin, BA, Mary Mullen, MS, and Sheilah Fish, MA, for their insights; Allure Jeffcoat, MS, a pioneer human sexuality college instructor and the person who gave me the opportunity to teach at the college level; and Diane Beeson, PhD, Juan Gonzales, PhD, and Kris Hammer, MA, for allowing me the pleasure of lecturing in their university and college classes.

Thank you to the many therapists who worked and supported me at the Relationship Counseling Center of Walnut Creek, California. Special thanks to Michael Tobin, PhD and Wes Laccoarce, MS—may their spirits be resting peacefully. And of course, not to forget the support and encouragement of Janet Forman, MA: my thanks.

Gratitude goes to Rosemary Gretton and Dan Cold, whose editorial work helped me turn content into readable English; and the publishing support of the team at Cognella (special thanks to Jessica Knott).

I appreciate my family's support, especially from my loving daughters, Danielle and Michelle Beaver, throughout this writing journey. My hope is that this book will help you experience intimate, healthy relationships.

Lastly, I want to thank Nancy Beaver, the best partner, friend, and wife a man could ever desire. Your love and support have given me the strength and conviction to write this book. You made it possible for me to take all my intellectual concepts and truly experience what it means to be intimate. I thought I knew before I met you, but I was wrong. Thanks for loving me for who I am. What a gift.

About the Author

A licensed Marriage and Family Therapist, Dan started his private practice in 1973 in Walnut Creek, California, and continues providing individual and couples therapy today. He co-founded the Relationship Counseling Center of Walnut Creek in 1974.

Dan is currently an instructor at Los Medanos College, Pittsburg, California where he teaches Psychology of Human Sexuality. He has also been a faculty member at J.F.K. University, CSU East Bay, and Diablo Valley College in Pleasant Hill, California.

The author of three books, *The Good Sex Bible*, *Creating the Intimate Connection*, and *Love Yourself*, Dan is also a popular speaker and presenter for education, business, and community groups.

Dan holds an M.S. in Counseling Psychology from California State University, East Bay and a B.A. in Psychology from University of California, Berkeley. He received specialized training in Masters and Johnson-style sex therapy, and has practiced as a sex therapist for over thirty years.

www.ingramcontent.com/pod-product-compliance
Ingram Content Group UK Ltd.
Pitfield, Milton Keynes, MK11 3LW, UK
UKHW061826190726
13853UKWH00009B/2461